Home Care Nursing Handbook

About the Author

Carolyn Humphrey, a home care nurse for nearly 20 years, is the Executive Director of the Visiting Nurse Association of the Valley in Derby, Connecticut. She received her Master's degree from the University of North Carolina School of Public Health and her Bachelor's degree from George Mason University. She earned her diploma in nursing at Kentucky Baptist Hospital in Louisville.

She has held nursing positions with the VNA in Washington, D.C. and with the Louisville Health Department. She was an Assistant Professor of nursing at Southern Connecticut State University and is an Adjunct Professor at the Yale University School of Nursing.

Home Care Nursing Handbook

Carolyn J. Humphrey, R.N., M.S.

APPLETON-CENTURY-CROFTS/Norwalk, Connecticut

Notice: The author(s) and publisher of this volume have taken
care that the information and recommendations contained
herein are accurate and compatible with the standards generally accepted at the time of publication.

Copyright © 1986 by Appleton-Century-Crofts
A Publishing Division of Prentice-Hall, Inc.

All rights reserved. This book, or any parts thereof, may not be
used or reproduced in any manner without written permission. For information, address Appleton-Century-Crofts, 25
Van Zant Street, East Norwalk, Connecticut 06855.

86   87   88   89   90 / 10   9   8   7   6   5   4   3

Prentice-Hall of Australia, Pty. Ltd., Sydney
Prentice-Hall Canada, Inc.
Prentice-Hall Hispanoamericana, S.A., Mexico
Prentice-Hall of India Private Limited, New Delhi
Prentice-Hall International (UK) Limited, London
Prentice-Hall of Japan, Inc., Tokyo
Prentice-Hall of Southeast Asia (Pte.) Ltd., Singapore
Whitehall Books Ltd., Wellington, New Zealand
Editora Prentice-Hall do Brasil Ltda., Rio de Janeiro

Library of Congress Cataloging-in-Publication Data

Humphrey, Carolyn J., 1947–
  Home care nursing handbook.

  Includes index.
  1. Home nursing—Handbooks, manuals, etc.
I. Title.   [DNLM: 1. Home Care Services—handbooks.
WY 39 H926h]
RT61.H86   1985   610.73′43   85–16599

ISBN 0-8385-3837-1

PRINTED IN THE UNITED STATES OF AMERICA

To the Public Health Nurse

"Many and varied are the duties which fall to the lot of the public health nurse. She often has to meet situations undreamed of by nurses in other fields."

To the Student Nurse

"As a student nurse practices caring for the sick, she comes to believe that the complicated and expensive equipment, such as is found in hospitals, is necessary for the simplest nursing procedure. This attitude is a great hindrance to effective work in the home care of patients and may prove very expensive to those she serves."

Lyla M. Olson, R.N.
Improvised Equipment in the Home Care of the Sick
W. B. Saunders Company, 1928.

Contents

Contributors

The following colleagues contributed in significant ways to the creation and reality of this handbook. Each brought her professional expertise and good humor in contributing to the sections of the book related to her specialty. All were willing to give constructive advice on the entire project while working on their own sections.

Dorothy Jacobson Baker, R.N.-C., M.N.
Assistant Professor, Yale University School of Nursing
Family Nurse Practitioner, Visiting Nurse Association, New Haven, Connecticut

Dorothy wrote the Physical Assessment Section in Chapter 2 and provided expert clinical comments and references to the entire manuscript. Her experiences in several agencies and as an advisor to students and practicing nurses provided the perfect mix of theory and practice.

Janice F. Goulet, R.P.T., M.S.
Therapy Coordinator
Visiting Nurse Association of the Valley
Derby, Connecticut

As a talented physical therapist, Janice developed the guidelines for referrals to all therapists in Chapter 1, the evaluation of functional assessment to determine referral to therapies in Chapter 2, and the various procedures and techniques relative to neurological patients in Chapter 3. She also contributed the section relative to homebound patients in Chapter 4.

Cheryl Tanner Marsh, M.S.N., R.N., C.S.
Psychiatric and Mental Health Clinical Nurse Specialist
Visiting Nurse Association of the Valley
Derby, Connecticut

Cheryl, a gerontology specialist, contributed the expertise and information found in Chapter 2—"Assessment of Psychological Functioning and Mental Status Assessment". Additionally, interventions relative to impaired cognitive functioning were developed from references and her clinical practice.

Paula Milone-Nuzzo, R.N., M.S.
Assistant Professor, School of Nursing
Southern Connecticut State University
New Haven, Connecticut

Paula brought many years of home care experience to the book and assisted with clarifying many aspects of the home visit in Chapter 1. She also wrote the content in Chapter 3 relative to interventions for the diabetic, cardiac, and thoracic patient. Her continuing encouragement and comments throughout the entire project were most valuable.

Eleanor Perrelli, R.N., B.S.N., E.T.
Enterostomal Therapist
Medical Sales Consultant
Hamden Surgical, Inc.
Hamden, Connecticut

Eleanor's experience as a home care nurse, an enterostomal therapist, and current work with a medical supply company proved very helpful throughout the handbook. She developed the section on interventions for the patient with impaired GI functioning and skin integrity found in Chapter 3, and provided many valuable references for review.

Nancy S. Suski, R.D.
VNA Nutrition Consultant
Regional Visiting Nurse Agency and
Visiting Nurse Association of New Haven
New Haven, Connecticut

Nancy combined her practical experience as a community health nutritionist and her sound educational background to write the guidelines for referring to a dietitian in Chapter 1, the nutrition assessment in Chapter 2, and all interventions relative to Diet—Nutrition found in Chapter 3.

My sincere thanks to each one.

Preface

This handbook will provide the home care nurse with a concise, compact guide that can be conveniently carried in the nurse's bag and used as a resource for those commonly found situations when more voluminous reference material is not accessible.

Home care nurses are generalists in a field of specialists. They are called upon every day to see different kinds of patients—patients in varying stages of diseases and illnesses—and with distinctive home environments and lifestyles. This handbook is intended to help the nurse remember the enormous amount of information needed to deliver care in the home.

Much of the information in this book comes from my 20 years of experience as a home care nurse, hospital and outpatient clinic nurse, teacher, and home care administrator. Additionally, practitioners in various fields contributed their expertise to the information presented in this handbook, and appropriate literature was reviewed.

Chapter 1 covers all aspects of the home visit including how to conduct the visit, determining visit frequency, what assessments indicate when a patient needs other services besides nursing, important reminders about recording information on the patient record, and guidelines on reimbursement, especially Medicare. Even though the material presented in this chapter is very helpful to the new home care nurse, the more experienced nurse can also benefit from periodically reviewing this section.

Chapter 2 includes various assessment guides to use when conducting visits on new or current patients. The guides for Health/Illness History, General Psychological Functioning, and Family Assessment should be used on all patients in determining initial information. The Physical Assessment section uses a head-to-toe review of systems and is set up in three columns—"how" to carry out a physical assessment; the "normal" section, that is, the normal parameters of assessment findings; and the "if abnormal" section which gives the nurse direction on when and how to intervene when deviations from normal are found.

The remainder of Chapter 2 provides more in-depth assessment guidelines in the areas of medication, nutrition, and psychological functioning. Also, two assessment questionnaires are given. The first measures a patient's ADLs so the nurse can better determine if a home health aide is necessary. The second is a scale that measures a patient's level of independent functioning to determine the need for physical, speech, and/or occupational therapy. The information presented in this chapter not only can be used for assessing need for service but also to assist in documenting pertinent information on the patient record.

Chapter 3 provides an outline of interventions based on the medical diagnoses most often found in home care. Not to be mistaken as a "cookbook approach" to nursing, the guidelines must be used in concert with professional judgment so appropriate interventions are chosen for the specific patient situation. Not only is the information helpful in describing possible ways to approach patient problems, but all interventions are written in care plan terminology that can be written directly on the patient record.

Chapter 4 outlines common home care procedures, techniques that often need to be taught to families and home health aides, patient teaching information, home preparation of solutions, and sterilization techniques.

Chapter 5, titled, "Helpful Hints and Improvised Equipment," includes those things home care nurses and patients learn from experience, *not* in textbooks! These hints and ideas for equipment can be valuable in providing cost effective care.

The Appendix has several reference charts that can be used for an in-depth review of specific information from earlier chapters and/or can be used when teaching patients. The Bibliography at the end of the handbook includes references used in the preparation of this handbook and books a home health agency or home care nurse may want as a library resource.

"Your Own Pages" are blank pages provided at the end of the book so the home care nurse can include specific community and agency information which can make this handbook a personal, useful tool. These handy sheets can be used for phone numbers, computer codes, and other information often necessary in the patient's home.

All chapters of the handbook include guidelines that can be used with all existing organizational forms and records: therefore, intentionally, no specific forms are given.

The word "family" has been used throughout this book to describe the support systems needed by the patient in the home and to stress the importance of the original basis of public health—family centered nursing. Since many elderly live alone, caregiver can be used interchangeably with the term family. Primary care provider can be substituted for the term physician when patients are seen by nurse practitioners in primary care clinics. Although there is some discussion of medications in each section of Chapter 3, it is important that the nurse use this handbook with an up-to-date comprehensive drug reference. The use, effectiveness, and side effects of drugs change frequently and the home care nurse must keep current.

I have written this handbook to assist the home care nurse in working with patients and families. It is to be used as a first resource, consulting more in-depth references whenever necessary. I hope this handbook will be helpful to home care nurses and students as a guide in delivering the wide scope of care that is demanded by today's home care nurse. By using practical, "common sense" coupled with professional, scientific knowledge, the home care nurse can be prepared to help the patient and family achieve the goals they mutually set.

Carolyn J. Humphrey, R.N., M.S.

Acknowledgments

The practicality and usefullness of this handbook is due greatly to the colleagues who have assisted me in its preparation. I have received input on all sections from individuals who not only have the scientific knowledge but the "hands on" experience that helped cull out the important aspects of home care.

First, many thanks go to Lazelle Benefield, R.N., M.S.N., who was able to take my disjointed conversations about home health care and form them into the original idea of this book.

Special thanks go to Mary Ellen K. Frele, R.N., M.B.A., Markat Health Management Consultants, who read the entire book and was generous with advice and support. I also appreciate the comments of Domenic A. Sammarco R.Ph., community pharmacist, who reviewed all material related to medications and Mary Ann O'Connor, R.N., B.S.N., Assistant Director of Trumbull Public Health Nursing, Trumbull, Connecticut, who reviewed Chapter 3 for clinical content.

Several individuals provided assistance at various times during the preparation of the text. I acknowledge the assistance of Connie Bove, R.N., M.S.; Irene Kalins, R.N., M.S.; and Gayle Bannon, R.N.

I am grateful to the management staff of the Visiting Nurse Association of the Valley as well as John Fiore, President of the Board. Their support allowed me to give this handbook the attention it deserved.

A thank you to Ann Moy, editor, for her words of encouragement, compassionate ear, and her belief in the concept of the book, and to Debbie Corson who patiently edited the manuscript.

A special thank you goes to Fred Gross whose support, understanding, expert editorial advice, and love have helped make this book a reality.

And finally, to all those patients and home care nurses I have been fortunate to work with during my career— thank you. You have taught me how to merge what I have learned in school with the lessons of life to become the person and nurse I am today.

1

Aspects of the Home Visit

In a hospital or nursing home, many areas dealing with the process of recovery or daily life are cared for without the patients' involvement. Special diets are prepared and brought to them on a regular basis. Medication is dispensed as ordered by the physician with the patient paying little thought to what it is for, how often it should be taken, or how to tell one little white pill from another.

Heat, electricity, and other environmental factors are controlled as are the personal care needs of the patient. Someone changes the bed every day and sees that there are towels. Transportation to physical, speech, and occupational therapy is arranged. The dietitian comes to the bedside to teach specifics about nutrition. Medical supplies and equipment are immediately available for patients. The hospital bill is usually paid for by a third party—an insurance company or a state agency. Even the physician stops in at least daily to see how things are going. This describes the situation in an institution: Not so in the home.

In the home, the patient or a family member has to take care of all these needs. How a patient copes with these needs often can only be determined by a home care nurse. Therefore, the home visit is an important aspect of the care provided by a home health agency.

The ability to conduct a successful home visit is an art that requires skills of clinical practice, counseling, communication, and psychology as well as expertise in cultural, social, and community assessment. Talking with the patient in their home environment gives the professional a unique opportunity to observe the many facets of the patient's life and how these facets affect health and illness.

Additionally, family members, friends, and neighbors can and should be included in the patient's assessment, plan of treatment, and evaluation. No matter how much detailed information a referral source gives concerning the patient, the home care nurse must always be receptive to the broader data base that will present itself during the home visit.

The various components of the home visit come together to create a dynamic picture of the patient. This picture can be used effectively by the home care professional in planning care. These components include: planning and conducting the visit, evaluating the need for services other than nursing, planning the specific care by using goal setting and contracting techniques, determining the reimbursement for care, making discharge plans, and, finally, recording the visit. These components are the focus of this chapter and are to be used as guidelines to assist the nurse in conducting the home visit.

Section I—Planning for the Visit

There are many steps in a home visit: each step should be implemented every time a visit is made. Depending on the kind of visit, that is, initial admission or follow-up visit, the steps are applied in varying degrees. A visit must be conducted in a logical progression so the nurse can use time efficiently and gather all information needed to develop a good plan of care.

In this section, the steps of a home visit will be outlined by "walking through" an initial visit. An initial visit is defined as that visit that establishes the foundation for future visits. It may be the first time a patient is seen by an agency, the first visit after a patient known to the agency is discharged from the hospital, or when a patient discharged from an agency at a previous time is readmitted for the same or a different problem.

Remember that it may take more than one visit to gather all information necessary to adequately plan for future care. Additionally, the home care nurse is assessing, planning, delivering, and evaluating care on *each* visit so the steps in the visit outlined in this section and Section II can be applied to initial and subsequent visits in varying degrees.

Preparation for the Visit

1. Determine the Purpose of the Visit: On an initial visit, the visit purpose can be determined by the written information on the referral and by the nurse's knowledge. There may be assessments that were made by the referring source that could lead to specific interventions. Additionally, the nurse's experience with similar patients assists in clarifying the purpose of the visit. On a follow-up visit, the goals of care determine the purpose for each visit.

2. Determine the Type of Visit to Be Conducted: On an initial visit, the focus is on assessing and developing a relationship with the patient and family as well as establishing the specific interventions that need to be implemented on subsequent visits. On follow-up visits, specific technical assistance, further assessment, or teaching can be at the center of the visit.

3. Set Priorities: Many patient situations are very complex, and several purposes for the visit arise simultaneously. Whether an initial or follow-up visit, the nurse should determine what needs to be done for the patient immediately and what can wait for future visits—whether this is in the area of assessment, intervention, or evaluation. Although the priorities are finally determined with the patient and family after a visit has been completed, focusing on priorities is important before making the initial visit.

4. Knowledge of the Patient and Family: Check on the patient's history and determine if the patient has been given service by the agency before. If so, review the patient's record and talk to others in the agency familiar with the case to learn significant information that will prepare you for the visit. Be careful not to get trapped into gossip or negative feelings that may be communicated from another staff member.

5. Check for Bias: Distinguish similarities and differences in the referral or visit from the kind of care the patient has received in the past. There may be a bias that is transmitted either from other staff in the agency or from the referring source that could "cloud" the important assessment information. Although the patient with a chronic disease can be admitted to a home health agency several times over many months or years, the professional needs to assure that each patient's admission to service is treated individually and that the observations of the patient are constantly reviewed and updated so appropriate care plans can be developed.

6. Call the Patient/Family: This call prepares the family for the nurse's visit psychologically and ensures that a family member will be at home if desired. Remember, the initial contact you make with the patient will set the tone for all future visits. If necessary, get directions to the house.

7. Previsit Precautions: Most agencies have policies governing the safety of staff. It is important to know the community to assure one's personal safety. No nurse, no matter how long she has worked in an area, should take her safety for granted and should review the following guidelines periodically. If there is any hesitancy at all about your own safety, either talk to the supervisor before the visit or call the supervisor if there are any concerns once the visit starts.

- Know exactly where you are going before you leave your office. Use a map. If you have any doubts about the location of a home, contact the family for directions. Leave a list of where you will be with your supervisor.
- Be certain to carry identification, including the phone numbers of the agency, police, and fire departments. The "Your Own Pages" Section in the back of this book has pages for these numbers.
- If you are driving, be sure that your car is in good working order and that you have sufficient gas. Always keep all doors locked. If you are taking public

transportation, be sure that you know your route. If you are walking, know your route and do not accept rides from anyone.

- Locking keys in the car can happen frequently. Consider either having a spare set in the nursing bag or keep keys in a magnetic holder hidden on the outside of the car.
- Do not carry excessive amounts of money with you. Do carry enough money for emergency transportation and phone calls.
- Avoid carrying a purse. If you carry a purse and are driving, lock it in your trunk before you leave the office and keep it there while visiting patients. A purse can be a temptation both on the streets and in homes; keep your money and identification in a pocket.
- Park as close to your destination as possible unless the home is in a potentially dangerous area; then park on a public street and walk the most direct route to the home.
- When walking, avoid groups of people lingering on corners or in doorways. Cross the street to avoid them.
- Carry keys in your hand. This will enable you to get into your car immediately and you can use them as a method of self defense. Hold the key ring in the palm of your hand and put one key between each of your four fingers with the sharp ends sticking out. You may also want to attach a whistle on your key ring which can be used if necessary to summon help.
- Dress appropriately. If you do not wear uniforms, wear conservative street clothes. Wear a name tag and carry some form of identification so patients can be assured you are a valid representative of the agency. Do not wear suggestive clothing. Wear shoes that fit comfortably and well so that you can move quickly and safely if necessary.
- If the agency policy is to travel in pairs, do so. This is not always a policy, nor is it always necessary. In some instances, it may be safer to take another nurse or escort on the visit. Check with the supervisor or another nurse that may know the area better.
- Never knock on unmarked doors or on the doors of

homes other than those of families whom you are visiting. Never walk into a home uninvited. Never enter
a vacant home.

- If there are any doubts about the safety of entering a
  home or apartment building, don't enter. Call the supervisor or return to the office.
- If walking in a densely populated area, walk in the
  middle of the sidewalk. Do not take short cuts down
  alleys, through buildings, or across private property.
  Avoid narrow or confined spaces.
- If a night visit must be made in a questionably safe
  area, local police often are willing to assist if you plan
  ahead and if the agency has no escort service.

(Adapted from: Burgess, Wendy, and E. Ragland, *Community Health Nursing: Philosophy, Process, Practice.*
Norwalk, Connecticut: Appleton-Century-Crofts, 1983. Used
with Permission.)

8. Read Appropriate Materials: Review aspects of the
disease process and possible interventions. Review medications, usual doses, side effects, and any other information that is relevant to the patient situation. Take any
patient information booklets needed to use as teaching
tools. Even though this is an initial visit, interventions
will still need to take place.

9. Check Supplies: Make sure that the patient has adequate supplies in the home for any procedures that need
to be done. Make sure that your nursing bag is well stocked.
The procedure for using the Nursing Bag follows.

THE NURSING BAG   The nursing bag has been the traditional symbol of home visiting since the turn of the cen-
tury. The type of nursing bag, standard equipment, and
procedure for use of the nursing bag vary from agency to
agency.

Although bag technique has often been laughed at as
"old fashioned," it remains an essential part of aseptic
technique that *must* be used in the home to prevent the
nurse from spreading pathogens from one patient to another. No matter how long a nurse has been practicing in
the community, a periodic review of bag technique is es-

sential so that bad habits are not formed which can endanger the patient and the nurse.

CONTENTS OF NURSING BAG   The equipment and supplies in the bag should include items the nurse will use daily on all patients. The nurse should think ahead to the type of service she is going to deliver that day and add any equipment to the bag for specific visits as necessary. The following supplies should be basic to all nursing bags:

1. Handwashing equipment—soap in plastic container and paper towels.
2. Assessment equipment—thermometers, stethoscope, a hem gauge to measure the size of wounds, sphygmomanometer, urine testing equipment.
3. Disposable supplies—plastic thermometer covers (if used in an agency), plastic aprons, sterile and nonsterile gloves, dressings, adhesive tape, alcohol swabs, tongue blades, applicators, lubricant jelly, scissors, Band-Aids, syringes and needles, and vacutainer equipment for venipuncture, if appropriate.
4. Paper Supplies—road map, new patient record, charge slips, any agency printed material needed to give to patient.
5. A copy of this book.

BAG TECHNIQUE   The following steps in bag technique should be used to maximize the efficient use of your bag and to assure that principles of asepsis are being carried out. Always explain to the patient and family why you are following a specified technique. They will look upon you as more professional and will be assured you have their safety uppermost.

1. Place the bag in a clean area, preferably on a wooden table. The bag should always be placed on something like a newspaper or paper towel to avoid contaminating the outside of the bag. Do not place your bag on stuffed furniture or at a level where an inquisitive child or pet could gain access to the bag and contaminate it or harm themselves. Always keep your bag in sight.

2. Select something that will be used to discard contaminated equipment such as a paper or plastic bag, or a bag made from newspaper.
3. *Wash your hands* with the soap and paper towels in the bag. It is always best to use your own soap and towels unless the patient has paper towels for your use. Do not use cloth towels unless the family has a clean one for your use only. Leave the equipment at the sink until the end of the visit.
4. Only now, after handwashing, can the nurse enter the bag and take out all the equipment needed for the visit. Place it on a clean paper towel.
5. Proceed with the visit and discard dirty equipment into the paper or plastic bag. Carefully dispose of the syringes so they cannot be reused and so no one gets stuck with a needle. If there is an unusually large, contaminated dressing, another bag may need to be used. The family should be taught how to discard all dirty equipment safely.
6. When the visit is completed, clean used equipment and *wash your hands* before replacing equipment in the bag. Never reenter the bag unless you have washed your hands.
7. Close the bag and leave it in the clean area until you are ready to leave.

Remember:

1. All items in the nursing bag are considered clean; therefore, the principles of asepsis must remain uppermost on the nurse's mind. When items are taken out and used with one patient, they should either be thrown away, if disposable, or cleaned before placing back in the bag to be used on another patient.
2. The floor is considered a "dirty" area—*never* put your bag on the floor (home, office, or car).
3. Newspapers are considered clean and can be used for several purposes in the home where more expensive items, such as, plastic trash bags, are not available.
4. Hand-washing supplies (soap and paper towels) are essential and should be placed on the top of the bag

so they can be used immediately upon reaching the patient's home. Remember, always wash your hands before starting the visit, and, again, at the end of the visit just before leaving the home.

5. When not in use, the bag should always be locked in a clean part of the trunk out of sight or taken indoors at the end of the day. Extreme heat and cold can damage equipment in the bag.

6. Do not bring the bag into particularly dirty homes or when the patient has a communicable disease. Prepare a small bag with soap, towels, and any other equipment you need for that specific visit. Include in that bag another clean paper bag in which to put back your cleaned equipment. At the end of the visit, return that equipment to your basic bag.

7. Use the patient's equipment whenever possible. This saves time in equipment preparation and cleanup and decreases the agency's cost per visit.

Section II—Steps In the Home Visit

1. Basic Information

The beginning social aspects of the home visit between the nurse and patient are very important since they set the stage for a mutually rewarding relationship between the patient and the agency. The nurse should always remember that she is a guest in the patient's home and should recognize that the setting and expectations are far different from those she personally experienced in the hospital. Additionally, the patient's home environment may be much different from her own home, and it is important to recognize and accept this so that effective nursing care can be given. Being careful not to track dirt and snow onto the carpet and asking permission to use the sink or go into the bedroom in search of medications are examples of how the nurse can communicate appropriate respect for the patient and the patient's home.

The basic information exchanged between the nurse and patient will be determined by the agency's specific forms. Information shared will become part of the patient's home health record and must be accurate. Information on the referral should be validated. The nurse should explain her role and describe the policies of the agency as they pertain to the patient.

2. Visit Precautions

Just as there are certain precautions every nurse should know and review frequently as visits are planned, other important measures should be kept in mind during a home visit to assure safety. If any of the situations listed here occur, the nurse should discuss the event with the supervisor to assure continuation of needed service. These are:

- If you have any fears about your safety during the visit, or if anyone in the house is drunk, do what is essential for the patient and leave.
- If any weapons are present, either ask that they be put away or leave. If you have any doubts, leave. If you are afraid to make such a request or have any doubts, leave.
- If a pet is particularly obnoxious to you or seems hostile, ask that it be put in another room or leave. Even if the pet doesn't seem hostile, when you begin to work with the patient the pet may perceive you are harming his master. Be sure to note on the record that there is an animal in the home who may be protective to the patient so others who visit the patient might take precautions. It is important, however, to be respectful of the patient's attachment to the pet at all times.
- Note all possible exits from the house should an emergency arise. Sit in such a way that you have easy access to these exits.
- Generally, do not take food from the patient or family. Explain that you are working and not able to eat or drink with them. Use discretion, ask if you can take the food with you—avoid comments the patient might find insulting.

(Adapted from Burgess, Wendy, and E. Ragland, *Community Health Nursing: Philosophy, Process, Practice.* Norwalk, Connecticut: Appleton-Century-Crofts, 1983. Used with Permission.)

3. Assessment

Specific areas of assessment are detailed in Chapter 3
and should be used in conducting this part of the visit.
Since the home care nurse has a unique opportunity to
care for the patient and family in their own home, it is
important that this assessment be implemented by using
the following techniques:

Interviewing—ask well-thought-out, relevant, open-
ended questions and listen carefully to the answers.
The patient/family should be doing most of the talking. Make notes or complete forms during the interview. If appropriate, share these forms with the patient or family for accuracy.

Observing—Objectively describe all areas of assessment including family relationships, atmosphere of
the home, and the patient/family's response to your
intervention.

Using Assessment Tools—The use of equipment such
as stethoscopes and thermometers in addition to specific assessment tools such as those found in Chapter
3 can enable you to develop baseline data. This data
is essential to the evaluation of the patient during
subsequent visits. Do not overlook the importance of
using all your senses, such as smell, touch, hearing,
and seeing, to fully assess the patient. Often judging
how a patient responds to a touch on the arm tells
you much about the entire situation such as suspicion,
fear of strangers, loneliness, and so on.

4. Planning the Interventions

After sufficient data about the needs of the patient and
family have been gathered, a plan of treatment is developed with the patient, family, physician, and other care
providers such as therapists, dietitians, and social workers. Suggestions for content of the plan of treatment based
on the impairment of the patient are found in Chapters 3
and 4 and will prove helpful in planning the specific interventions. These interventions cannot be used successfully unless the nurse is involved with goal setting and

applies principles of contracting to her work with patients and families.

Goal setting and contracting are important concepts that must be understood in setting up the interventions for each patient. The emphasis on goal setting and contracting in home care makes delivering care in the home different from planning care in an institutional setting. To assist the home health nurse in applying these principles to practice, the following aspects of goal setting and contracting are outlined.

Goal Setting   Based on the assessment of the patient, family, and environment gathered during the home visit, the information on the referral, and the nurse's knowledge of the situation, short- and long-term goals should be established. The following principles should be used when setting goals:

A. **Goals should always be realistic, measurable, and achievable for the patient.** Goals of care that the nurse views as important must be discussed openly with the patient and family. The goals the patient and family wish to accomplish through working with the home health agency should be elicited and weighed heavily in planning care.

B. **Goals should be outcome oriented.** Outcome-oriented goals focus attention on the end results of care. They are written to measure behavioral change within the patient rather than the process nurses use to effect the patient change. They focus on what a patient has learned, for example, not on what or how a nurse has taught specific information. By clarifying desired outcomes with the family and patient, it is easier to determine how a patient is to reach the established goals as service is being given. In addition, outcome-oriented goals also clearly identify when the patient is ready for discharge since the goals, mutually established, have been achieved. This prevents the patient and/or family from being negatively "surprised" that the home health agency is discharging the patient.

C. **Goals should be listed in order of priority and readjusted as needs and situation dictates.** In the home setting, many patient problems, each with relative goals, arise at one time. Short-term goals should focus on the main problem; long-term goals are identified, but they can be "put on the back burner" for a later time. Each goal should be attainable by a certain time frame, which can range from a few days to a few months depending on the nature of the care required. Each goal should include a statement indicating a time estimate for when the goal can be reached.

Contracting   Webster's Dictionary defines a contract as an agreement between two or more people to do something. In contrast to legal contracts, which are written and binding agreements, the contract in a helping relationship should be clear to both parties while remaining flexible and should be based on a clear understanding of the goals and the *way* the goals are to be accomplished.

Although a contract is usually a written document, a contract used in home care nursing practice should at minimum be a verbal agreement that ties into the goal setting process just listed. A nurse may feel the contract needs to be written, or agency policy may dictate such practice in certain situations. Basically, a home care nurse's contract with a patient and family is a working agreement that outlines exactly what the nurse, family, and patient are to do in the situation. This agreement is known to both parties and can be continuously renegotiated.

Contracting by the home care nurse is essential to the success of all care given to patients in the home. The relationship between a patient and a nurse in the home environment is much different and often more critical than in an institution such as a hospital or nursing home. Procedures that professional nurses carry out for the patient in the hospital are not always done in the home directly by the nurse, but instead they are taught to the patient and family so both patient and family can be more independent. Additionally, the way in which procedures and therapeutic regimes are carried out in the home must be modified to the specific environment and patient situation. These different role expectations can lead to major misunderstandings among all home health agency personnel, patients, and family unless clarified during the initial visit with contracting.

MAIN FEATURES OF CONTRACTING:

1. **Partnership.** All aspects of the contract with patients involve shared participation and agreement; the patient and the health provider become partners in the relationship.
2. **Commitment.** Both parties make a decision that binds them to fulfilling the purpose of the contract; it is a pledge of trust in the nurse and dedication to the goal.
3. **Format.** By setting a contract, both the patient and nurse obtain a clear idea of the purpose of the relationship, of their respective responsibilities, and of the specific limits within which they will work. Once a contract is established, *what* has to be done, *who* is to do it, and *within* what time frame is clear.
4. **Negotiation.** Contracting with patients always involves negotiation. A period of give and take and suggestions on how to best reach the goal are shared constantly between the parties.

A CONTRACT BETWEEN THE AGENCY AND THE PATIENT INCLUDES:

1. A thorough understanding of the plan of care needed to accomplish the goals by all involved. This plan includes the *specific* activities that need to be carried out and by whom. Although the plan can be altered on the basis of what happens in the future, the nurse must be clear with herself and the patient/family on exactly what things need to be done.
2. Expectations of the Patient/Family. Critical to setting a contract is a discussion and clarification of the roles and expectations of all involved. Often patients think nurses have all the answers and are fearful of sharing their thoughts and feelings. If this is not dealt with initially in the relationship, the entire interactions and plan of care can be negatively impacted.
3. An outline of the specific procedures and responsibilities each member of the home health agency will assume as well as what exactly will be expected from the patient and family. Agencies should have written guidelines, such as "A Patient Bill of Rights and Re-

sponsibilities," that outline not only the rights of the patient but the role and responsibilities the patient and family must assume to receive the intermittent care provided by the home health agency.

4. A specific time frame for carrying out the contract. This includes the expected frequency of visits to be made by the home health agency team, when the plan should be reevaluated, and the interaction of the nurse with the patient's physician. In some cases, it is also appropriate to outline in the contract the anticipated time period for reimbursement of care. Knowing that financial support is limited often helps the patient take the entire experience more seriously and focus on reaching the goals since the assistance from the agency is limited.

Benefits of Contracting   By developing a plan through the use of goal setting and contracting, the roles and expectations of everyone are clarified. Carrying out the treatment plan will be much easier because:

1. The patient is involved in his own care.
2. Setting specific measurable goals motivates patients to perform necessary tasks.
3. Care plans can be individualized by focusing on the patient's unique needs.
4. The possibility of reaching the goals are increased because all parties are clear on what the goals are.
5. Problem-solving skills of both the nurse and patient are developed.
6. The patient becomes an active partner in the decision-making process relative to his self-care.
7. The patient's autonomy and self-esteem are heightened as they learn self-care.
8. The service of the nurse, as well as others on the health team, is used more efficiently, and care becomes more cost effective.

Intervention   Interventions occur to a lesser extent on the initial visit than on subsequent visits. Most interventions that occur on the initial visit are task oriented, preliminary teaching, or gathering more information. This is not to say that the nurse should not be as efficient as possible and cover intervention on the first and second visit, if appropriate. Specific aspects of intervention and evaluation related to various impairments are outlined relative to specific diagnoses and impairments in Chapter 3.

Determining Frequency of Visits   On the initial visit as well as subsequent visits, the nurse must decide how frequently a patient needs to be seen. The frequency of visits is based on the physician's orders and the nurse's judgement of the condition of the patient as well as any state, federal, or agency policy. The following list is to be used as a guideline to assist the nurse in determining frequency of visits. If a patient requests more service than the physician or nurse feels is needed, agency policy and procedures should be consulted.

Patients Who Need to be Seen the Next Day:

1. Nurse has an incomplete data base on which to make a judgement and needs to obtain more data the next day.
2. Immediate teaching needs or subject matter of teaching is so complex it must be divided into smaller segments.
3. The patient's condition is unstable, and a serious change in the patient's condition could potentially occur.
4. The complex procedure requires a skilled professional to administrate.
5. Physician's orders need to be specifically followed.
6. The family is having serious difficulty coping with the patient at home and needs teaching (for management as well as further assessment for additional support).
7. While searching for caregiver who can be taught procedure such as, insulin injections, dressing changes.

Next Visit—Two to Three Days:

Note, this should be the *minimum* of time between the initial and subsequent visit.

1. Monitoring of condition that needs short-term follow up.

2. To implement and reinforce teaching plan.
3. To evaluate the effect of treatment plan (that is, medication, procedure, diet).

Weekly:

1. Patients who need minimal monitoring.
2. When needed to perform specified treatments.
3. To evaluate entire teaching plan toward end of time on service.
4. For evaluation of family's coping ability and use of other agencies if applicable.

Monthly and Longer:

1. Patients who are at optimal level of care.
2. Specific orders for treatments or monitoring on a monthly basis.
3. To measure compliance or effect of teaching/learning.
4. To fulfill regulations or compliance with reimbursement guidelines.

5. Closing the Visit

Ending a visit, especially the initial one, is extremely important since it clarifies what is to be expected in future encounters and establishes the relationship between the nurse and agency with the patient and family. During all visits it is important to include these items when ending a visit:

1. Give a brief review of the main points you have made.
2. Stress the positive behaviors identified and patient/family strengths.
3. Reiterate the teaching plan and plan of treatment; explain what you and/or someone else will do on the next visit. *Be sure the* patient knows who the primary care nurse is. Major points should be put in writing and left with the patient.
4. Discuss the frequency of visits by all anticipated personnel based on the outcome of this day's visit (*see* "Determining Frequency of Visit," page 16).
5. Be sure the patient has your name and knows how

to reach you at your office. *Do not give out your home phone number in any situation.*
6. Set a day, date, and time for the next visit.

6. Evaluation of the Visit

After each home visit the nurse should ask herself:

1. Are the patient, family, and I in agreement regarding the purpose and objective of the visit and service?
2. Have I been able to measure the family's understanding of my teaching plan?
3. Is there a measurable difference in the patient or family's understanding because of the visit today?
4. Does the patient's record indicate in a clear, concise manner what transpired on this home visit?
5. Do I need to seek other opinions or other resources to better care for this patient?
6. Do I need to report any deviations in my assessment to the physician?
7. Does my entire plan show continuity and a long-term plan that indicates when the patient will be discharged from service?
8. Is there anything I would do differently the next time I face such a situation?

As the nurse ponders the answers to these questions the supervisor should be consulted if questions arise that need clarification. By taking the small amount of time needed to evaluate her clinical performance, the appropriateness of the plan of care, and the patient's compliance with it, the nurse will continue to provide the best care.

7. Subsequent Visits

A thorough initial assessment that leads to a sound plan of treatment makes subsequent visits easier and more productive. Since the home visit is like the art of nursing—a dynamic, changing process—the steps in the home visit outlined in the previous pages are implemented with varying emphasis each time a home visit is made. Throughout subsequent visits the nurse should continue to evaluate the effectiveness of the plans made and look for new problems that may only reveal themselves with time and familiarity.

8. Discharging a Patient from Service

The discharge of a patient from service should be planned from the initial visit. When the frequency of visits, reimbursement source, and need of the patient are outlined in the contract, the time of discharge becomes evident to the patient and the nurse. Thus, the discharge of the patient can be smoothly handled. Other situations also arise that indicate a patient must be discharged from the home health agency.

Criteria for Discharge from Home Care

1. The goals for the patient set out in the contract have been achieved.
2. The patient may or may not be homebound.
3. The care (nursing, physical, or speech therapy) required by the patient need no longer be skilled.
4. The patient is hospitalized and time of return to the home is unknown.
5. The patient refuses further service by the agency.
6. The patient moved or is moving out of the service area of the agency.
7. The service now needed for the patient is not available from the home health agency.
8. No funding is available to provide the care.
9. The patient expired.
10. The home situation is unsafe, and intermittent care is not adequate to meet the patient's needs satisfactorily. In this situation, agency policies should be consulted to address issues of abandonment.

Although all of these situations are applicable for discharge, at times a patient desires to continue receiving home services, on a private pay basis. If this is the case, the nurse should consult the agency's policies.

Discharge Summary   Although agencies have varying requirements and formats for recording the patient's discharge from a home health agency, the following basic procedures should be carried out and recorded when a patient is discharged from service:

1. If possible, two weeks before the planned discharge, the nurse should begin discussing discharge with the patient and family.
2. All care providers in the agency, as well as the physician, should discuss the plans for discharge.
3. A discharge visit should be made so the nurse can accurately assess the patient's condition upon discharge from the agency. A patient should always be discharged through a visit; never discharge a patient over the phone.
4. The entire patient's record should be brought up to date, including how the agency's procedure for discharge was implemented.
5. The Discharge Summary should show: the patient's condition at discharge, the reason for discharge (items 1-10, page 19), and plans for any future care. This part of the record should be as its name implies—a summary of all care the patient has received from time of admission to the agency, his reaction to the care, and the outcome of the service. Again, the discharge summary must relate to the goals and contract.

Section III—Evaluation for Other Services

As the person who develops the plan of treatment, the home care nurse is responsible for assessing the patient's need for services provided by other disciplines. Often the referring source or physician indicates the specific services desired; but, most often the nurse makes the final determination of which disciplines to consult after the initial home visit.

When to Refer to Other Services

All referrals to other services should arise from a need for assessment, for teaching of patients and/or caregivers, and/or for providing a specific treatment or service to the patient.Medicare coverage for therapy services also deals with the level of complexity necessary (*see* page 28, "Reimbursement Sources for Home Care").

The following guidelines can be used by the nurse to determine what other services might be needed by the patient. Although many agencies do not have all the services listed below, the lists overlap in many areas so that an appropriate discipline can usually be contacted.

Physical Therapy   A physical therapist should be consulted when:

1. The patient has an inability to ambulate safely.
2. The patient/family are unable to successfully perform transfers safely and effectively.
3. A home assessment for safety and/or modification in the home is needed.
4. An assessment of the need for assistive devices or instruction in their use is needed.
5. The patient's mobility status has changed significantly.
6. The patient's balance and coordination is a problem.
7. The patient has a loss of function of one or more extremities either by loss of range of motion (ROM) or strength.
8. The patient needs restorative therapy.
9. There is an exacerbation of a chronic disease causing decreased physical functioning.
10. The patient has an impairment in cardiac status and functioning and needs cardiac rehabilitation.
11. The patient has an impairment in pulmonary functioning requiring postural drainage and teaching.
12. The patient needs special physical therapy modalities, such as, ultrasound or neurostimulation.
13. The home health aide needs to be instructed in proper techniques for assistive care as specific to a patient.
14. The patient's caregivers need instruction in proper body techniques to safely care for the patient.
15. The patient's caregivers need instruction on the easiest and most efficient ways to meet the patient's activities of daily living.

Occupational Therapy   Occupational Therapy can be consulted when the patient has an *impairment* of:

1. The ability to conduct self care and activities of daily living (ADL) skills
2. Motor function of the upper extremities that resulted in decrease in strength and range of motion
3. Fine motor skills
4. Sensation
5. Cognitive and perceptual motor abilities
6. Cognitive mental status to implement reality orientation planning program
7. Body image
8. Communication skills mainly in the areas of writing, using the telephone, and making their needs understood.

Occupational therapy can also be used when:

9. The patient has difficulty with joint inflammation and pain and needs to be taught joint protection techniques and pain management skills and needs to be evaluated for supportive devices such as splints or slings.
10. The patient has an easy onset of fatigue and limited mobility secondary to shortness of breath (SOB) and needs to be taught energy conservation.
11. Assessment is needed to eliminate physical barriers to better adapt the home environment, for example, kitchen adaptation.

Speech Therapy   A speech therapist can be consulted when the patient exhibits the following symptoms:

1. Loss or impairment of communication skills as indicated by a change in communication (expressive, receptive).
2. Muscular loss or weakness in facial or throat areas.
3. Loss of phonation, such as after a laryngectomy or other surgical procedures.
4. Changes in receptive or expressive abilities such as:

   a. difficulty following directions
   b. confusion
   c. negativity
   d. unresponsiveness

  e. inappropriate responses
  f. consistently communicates with one- or two-word responses
  g. perseveration of speech

5. Memory deficits.
6. Reading, writing, or visual difficulty.
7. Verbal and Oral Apraxia—inability to carry out the verbal act.
8. Inadequate use of gestures.
9. Neurological impairment secondary to the disease process.
10. Cognitive or language disorders.
11. Hearing loss.

Enterostomal Therapy Enterostomal therapists, some-time called Ostomy Specialists or E.T.s, have broadened their scope of practice to include other areas than just the management of ostomies. If you have a patient with any of the following situations you should refer the patient and/or consult directly with an available E.T.

1. Problems with ostomy management
2. Incontinency—urine or fecal
3. Problems with skin integrity, such as decubitus care or wound management

Nutritionist or Dietitian Home health agencies should have access for staff consultation with a dietitian. Many situations arise that require a broad knowledge base of diet therapy and nutritional requirements beyond the scope of basic nursing. The following situations are indicative of times when a nutritionist should be consulted.

1. A complete nutrition assessment is required.
2. When the patient and/or family require teaching and clarification of complex regimes.
3. Therapeutic diets need to be adapted to lifestyle patterns or ethnic or cultural eating habits.
4. Changes in diet orders are made that require computation and adaptation of the existing diet therapy.
5. When the patient fails to accept nursing interventions to intercept declining nutritional status.
6. When an additional opinion may help with the eval-

uation of problems related to eating or nutrient intake.

Social Services   Referrals to social services and social
workers are usually dependent on the specific responsibilities given to these services in the home health agency.
The most frequent referrals are:

1. Ongoing/intense involvement with other agencies and
   resources in the community
2. Assistance regarding patient financial matters
3. Counseling provided in the home for patients and
   families
4. Intervening directly for the patient/family and/or nurse
   with community resources.

Home Health Aide   Home health aides (HHAs) can provide essential assistance to the homebound patient and
respite for family members. The care given by the aide
includes assisting the patient with ADLs as well as specific
procedures that are supervised by the nurse or therapist.
Guidelines for determining requirements for HHAs should
be used in collaboration with the services desired by the
patient and agency policy regarding use, responsibilities,
and reimbursement.

Determining the need for a home health aide requires
the evaluation of two variables: the patient's degree of
independence and mental status. An in-depth discussion
of *how* to assess a patient's mental status and Activities
of Daily Living is found in Chapter 2. This information
can be used to assist the nurse in determining the need
for placement of a home health aide, documenting the care
given, and teaching the aide the specific tasks necessary
for the patient.

The patient and family must understand the limits of
reimbursement for HHA service and any other available
agency resources and/or affordable alternative which provides other levels of care. Often, patients and families can
become dependent on the HHA service and when it is
withdrawn have a more difficult time than before the aide
was placed. Try to prevent this from happening through
the use of contracting, goal setting, and explaining reimbursement issues fully.

The Medicare regulations pertaining to reimbursement for home health aide service can be used as guidelines for all placements unless specific agency or state regulations supersede. These are:

1. The patient must require skilled nursing, physical therapy, or speech therapy.
2. The HHA must give personal care in addition to cooking and/or care of the environment if necessary.
3. The order for a HHA must be renewed every sixty (60) days.
4. The continued need for an aide must be documented frequently, *at least* every two weeks.
5. The initial aide visit to the patient should be made with the primary care nurse responsible for the patient.
6. The nurse and/or therapist is responsible for controlling the assignment and directing care with the family.
7. The HHA must be supervised every two weeks by the primary care nurse. It cannot be stressed enough that the primary care nurse is responsible for supervising the HHA in the patient's home. Understanding this responsibility and reflecting when and how this requirement is accomplished is essential to placement of a HHA. Essential components of HHA supervision are:

- A clear description of why HHA service is needed and how it relates to the care goals.
- The HHAs acceptance by the patient and family. How are they reacting to the the presence of the HHA? Use observed behaviors.
- The plan for the direct care and assistance to be given. This must be *specific* and complete. Agencies have plans of instructions that should be fully completed for each patient.
- The plan for long-term independence. This should have been addressed in goal setting and contracting when the time for the HHA's service has been estimated.
- The alternate resources that allow the HHA to be an augment to other assistance the patient may need.

- The HHA's role in teaching independence. Any specific goals aimed at fostering patient's independence.
- Safety factors in the home. How safe the situation is while the HHA is in the home and when no agency personnel are present. What specific items is the HHA to observe for, and how and to whom is she to report?

Referral to Other Agencies   When the nurse finds that patient problems or family situations can more appropriately be handled by other agencies or providers, the patient and family should be referred to an agency that can be helpful. Since the patient relies on the nurse's judgement regarding the reliability of the agency, it is important that the nurse follow up on referrals periodically to see what patients think of the agency. It is also important that she establish a relationship with a contact person at frequently used agencies so referrals can be expedited, and patients can get more personalized care. Referring should always be done with the consent of the patient and the family; the reason for the referral should be clear and mutually agreed upon.

After receiving permission from the patient to contact an agency on their behalf, the referral process can be expedited by transmitting the following information about the patient to the referring agency:

1. Name, address, phone number, and date of birth.
2. Name, address, phone number, and relationship of a close relative or friend.
3. The employer. If not employed or retired, an overview of the patient's financial situation, that is, amount and source of income, savings, other financial resources.
4. The name of the physician and of someone who can be notified in case of emergency.
5. If the patient has been seen by the agency before, and if so, when and for what reason.
6. The reason for the referral, stating the center of the problem including what kind of help the patient wants as well as your opinion of what is needed.
7. The name of all other agencies working with this patient.

Section IV—Reimbursement Sources for Home Care

It is important to clarify with patients the source of payment for services. After the assessment you will have a better idea of the services they will need, and you will be ready to discuss how the services can be reimbursed. An outline of the most common fee sources for home health care follows.

Private Insurance

Many private insurance companies have some coverage for home health depending on the specific policy carried individually by the patient and/or the company for which they work. Sometimes a patient may have more than one health insurance company. If this is the case, information should be gathered on *all existing policies* so fee determination can be made to give the patient the benefit of the best coverage possible through the various companies.

When working with private insurance carriers, all pertinent information must be collected by the nurse to facilitate the handling of payments. The nurse must obtain the following information from the patient:

1. Name of all health insurance companies
2. The identification number of the patient
3. Name of insured, if other than the patient
4. The contact person's telephone number and address at the insurance company or at place of employment
5. If the insurance company is not one familiar to the agency, a copy of the policy may need to be obtained for the business office to review and validate for home care coverage. This will be based on individual agency's policies.

Medicare

Medicare is a health insurance program of the federal government administered through the Department of Human Services by the Health Care Financing Administration (HCFA). Medicare was established through the Social Security Act and is funded by the Federal Government with only a small premium paid by individuals. Beneficiaries pay a deductible once a year on Part A (Hospital Care) and another on Part B (outpatient services and DME—durable medical equipment). If the patient is covered by Medicare they should have a Medicare card. It is important to check their complete Medicare number. Criteria for Medicare coverage of home visiting changes frequently but the five (5) eligibility criteria are outlined here:

1. The service must be skilled   Service must be provided under the supervision of a registered nurse, physical therapist, or speech therapist. For each specific service, coverage can be received for:

Nursing

- Dressings, irrigations
- Teaching, training
- Observation
- Medication administration

Physical Therapy (PT)

- Restorative therapy
- Gait training
- Ultrasound, Diathermy
- Therapeutic exercises

Speech Therapy (ST)

- Restorative therapy
- Diagnostic and evaluation services
- Therapeutic services, that is, patients with CVA, neurological diagnoses, laryngeal cancer

Nursing, physical, and speech therapy are the only services Medicare denotes as skilled; therefore, at least one must be essential for the patient to be reimbursed through Medicare. Additional services can be provided as long as there is one skilled service (nursing, PT, or ST) needed by the patient. These additional services and conditions for coverage are:

Occupational Therapy (OT)

- Restorative therapy for improving patient's function

- Designing, fabricating and fitting of orthotic and self-help devices
- Teaching of compensating techniques
- Designing a maintenance exercise program

Medical Social Services

- M.S.W. intervention must contribute significantly to the treatment of a patient's medical condition
- Indicated when social problems impede the progress or stability of patient's medical condition

Home Health Aide Service

- Personal care duties
- Semiskilled aspects of patient care, such as, assisting with exercise program
- Plan of care must be established by an R.N.
- Housekeeping service, such as changing linens and doing laundry, must be minimal
- Service should be medically necessary and justifiably linked to the disease and individual plan of care

2. The patient is homebound

- The patient has a condition which restricts his ability to leave his place of residence
- Leaving home would require a considerable and taxing effort
- Assistance of another person necessary to leave home
- Use of supportive devices necessary to leave home
- Special transportation necessary
- Absences from home are infrequent and of very short duration

3. The level of care must be part-time and intermittent

- There is a medically predictable recurring need
- There is a reasonable expectation that the patient's condition will change within a limited time-frame
- The frequency of service must be determined by specific needs of the patient and may be from as much as daily to as little as every 90 days in the case of

patients with silicone catheters. The nurse must justify the reasons the service is necessary and the frequency and keep current on agency and Medicare policy regarding the application of the definition of part-time and intermittent.

4. There must be an original plan of treatment authorized by an M.D. with a recertification every sixty (60) days   The *original* plan of treatment must include:

- The types of services required and their frequencies
- A long-range forecast of likely changes in the patient's condition
- The diagnosis—not the symptoms
- Functional limitations
- Certification of homebound status
- List of current medications
- The current diet
- The medical supplies necessary

The *Recertification* must include:

- Why there is a need for continuation of service
- The care provided is still reasonable and necessary
- That care is acute, not chronic/custodial
- The level of care required has not changed

5. The care is medically reasonable and necessary

- Plan of Care must reflect what is clinically wrong with the patient
- What each service will accomplish for the patient must be clear (goal setting should be clear)
- The outcomes for the patient must be clearly identified
- The time-frame established for the care must be clear
- The expectations for the patient must be realistic
- The entire plan of treatment must correlate with the patient's medical problems

Patients and nurses are often confused about what is covered by Medicare. Therefore, it is imperative that the home care nurse understand what is covered and how it is applied to the patient's care and explain this thoroughly to the patient and family. If questions arise which cannot be answered immediately, you should refer to the Medicare manual (HM11) and consult with the supervisor before any final payment plan is determined for the patient.

Planning for a patient's discharge from home care should be initiated on the admission visit. The patient and family should know what Medicare covers and when and how payment is denied. If appropriate, the patient and family should be informed of the patient's right to the appeal process.

Medicaid (Title 19)

Medicaid is a medical assistance program that is jointly administered by each state and the federal government. It is not an insurance program but an assistance program to help families with dependent children, the aged, blind, or disabled persons who cannot pay for health care because of limited financial resources. It is also intended to furnish rehabilitation and other services to help families and other individuals attain or retain capacity for independence of self care.

Unlike Medicare, each state develops its own health care service program under Medicaid. Since this variable exists, the nurse must be aware of specific policies governing Medicaid payments for home health in the state and agency policy regarding coverage. State welfare numbers and cards should be validated on admission and periodically depending on each state's and agency's policies.

Other Fee Sources

Some agencies have numerous other fee sources that can be used to provide services to patients. The nurse should be aware of these. You can use the section of this book, titled "Your Own Pages," to record specific information about these sources for your handy reference.

Section V—Recording the Visit

Every home health agency has its own form and style for recording information on a patient's chart. All agency personnel should remember that the chart is a legal and permanent record of the care given to the patient. The chart is used to decide if the care was appropriate and reimburseable. Even though recording formats and requirements vary from state to state and agency to agency, certain guidelines for documentation apply to all agencies.

Reimbursement for home health care is based on an illness model that requires documentation to justify specific patient care. Although most of the guidelines that follow are applicable to Medicare patients, they can be used when documenting care for other pay sources as well. Whether your agency uses a SOAP (subjective, objective, assessment, and planning) format or one of the many others available, the following hints and suggestions can be used to assure that care given is documented appropriately for all patients.

General Tips

1. Always record the day, month, year, and, if appropriate, time of the visit on *all* entries.
2. Since patients, reimbursement, and legal entities have access to charts, do not chart any judgements that can be interpreted by the patient or a court as discriminatory.
3. Try not to label people: Describe only behaviors that are observed and help patients clarify labels they give themselves. Then the record can indicate exactly what the patient said rather than a subjective, vague label. For example, depression is a label that is too often given to patients without specific observed behaviors such as affect, response, and so on listed in the record. The observations made by the nurse that indicated the patient was depressed and the feelings and symptoms recounted by the patient should be recorded so that an appropriate diagnosis can be made by someone legally able to diagnose.
4. Remember, conclusions or opinions are not acceptable in a court of law. Your value system comes into play in situations, for example, something "filthy" by your standards could be "clean" by the standard of others—describe the situation as it is.

5. Write legibly. Even though handwriting may be beautiful, if it isn't easily read, you and the agency could be in danger of misinformation and increased use of time to answer queries from reimbursement sources. Use definitions and abbreviations approved by your agency.
6. When making corrections always mark through information with one line and then date and initial the correction.

Remember: Never erase or use white out on any part of the chart.

Recording on the Care Plan and Narrative

The care plan is the guide to all patient care given by the agency and the progress note, sometimes called the narrative, embellishes what is written elsewhere in summary form. Not only is a complete documentation of the comprehensive care plan important for reimbursement and legal issues, it is also critical to the evaluation of competent nursing practice used in quality assurance.

As stated earlier, since most care provided by a home health agency is care of the sick, the documentation should be noted on the negative, that is, illness thus focusing on the statement of the problem(s) and the skilled care provided to deal with the problem(s). While progress is important to note, it is equally important to note the remaining unstable nature of the patient.

General Guidelines for Both the Care Plan and Progress Notes

1. Remember, you are taking a picture of a patient at a specific point in time. This "snapshot" is used not only to assess the patient's current status but also as a base of information to evaluate future changes.
2. With this "snapshot" in mind, do not record judgements even when describing objective findings such as physical assessment data. Statements like "within normal limits" and appetite "good" not only give little information about the description of the pa-

tients current status, but mean absolutely nothing when used as a baseline for comparisons in the future.

Guidelines for the Care Plan

1. The care plan should address all care delivered to the patient on the basis of all identified problems, not just the ones that focus on the primary diagnosis.
2. The care plan must reflect problems complex enough to require skilled care.
3. Goals should be identified clearly with nurse-and patient-centered actions listed below so implementation of the plan is clear.
4. If flow sheets are used, the care plan should be concise so each line of the flow sheet is easily followed.

Guidelines for the Progress Notes

1. Every note *must* stand alone.
2. Progress notes should periodically indicate homebound status.
3. The note must reflect all observations (both objective and subjective).
4. The note must state clearly and concisely the specific skilled interventions used to resolve the problem(s). Teaching and involvement of the family in the plan of care should always be stressed.
5. The note should reflect the reaction of the patient/family to all interventions, especially the success of the teaching plan.
6. The note should include description of any staff that were supervised in the home and evaluation of that personnel; include your review with input from the patient and family.
7. The note should conclude with the goal(s) the nurse plans to achieve with future nursing interventions and the rationale for any increase or decrease in frequency of visits.
8. The note should reflect any psychosocial changes occurring in the family.

Specific Tips on Charting

1. Rarely use the words "stable, plateau, independence, or maintenance" unless used in the context of explaining the remaining unstable aspects of the patient's condition. The word stable should only be used when the patient is ready to be discharged.
2. Always explain why trips outside the home are taken. Since homebound status is important in home care, the patient usually only leaves the home for activities related to therapy or physician's appointments.
3. Don't record the amount of the wound healed, record the amount yet to heal. On the record make sure the size of the wound is noted with measurement, that is, inches or the size of a quarter, color, drainage, and odor.
4. Don't write that family or patient is unwilling to learn the procedure. If there is a psychological problem with coping or comprehension, document that specifically for it reinforces the continued need for skilled care to address the problem. This situation is an excellent one to refer to a social worker or psychiatric nurse whose care is more easily seen as reimburseable in this case.

The Physician's Plan of Treatment

Although initial orders for home health services come from the physician, most agencies send back to the patient's physician a more complete order sheet based on the nurse's assessment and pertinent patient information relative to the home. The format and content of the Physician's Plan of Treatment (PPOT) vary on the basis of state, federal, or agency regulations but should include at least the following information:

1. Client and M.D. identifying information
2. Diagnoses, both primary and secondary, with the dates of onset
3. An establishment of homebound status under functional limitations
4. The current diet and medication regime

   5. The rehabilitation potential and goal(s)
   6. Specific orders that meet the total client needs

When to Change a Plan of Treatment

1. When a change in the patient's condition results in changes in the plan of treatment.
2. When the patient is hospitalized and returns to the home health agency upon discharge.
3. When there is a change in the support the patient is receiving from a caregiver, family member, and/or community agency.
4. For Medicare, every 60 days from date of admission to service.

Remember: When communicating with the physician, either in writing or verbally, report on the patient in a systematic way from head to toe as outlined in the assessment chapter. Physicians think this way and you will be better able to communicate your information in a successful way.

Recording the Telephone Encounter

Often the nurse implements part of the care plan through the telephone. Whether this is to the patient, family, physician, or other agency, this "encounter" must be documented accurately in the record. A telephone encounter should record:

1. The date and time of the contact and who specifically was talked to.
2. The reason for the contact and who contacted whom.
3. The information transmitted to the contact person. This can be a general statement referring to the specific information found elsewhere in the record.
4. A summary of the outcome including what specific message was received from the contact person and what decisions were made.
5. A note of what was done with the information received, that is, the patient contacted with the information received, documented elsewhere in the record, and so on.
6. The nurse's signature and title.

2

Assessment Guidelines

Patient assessment in the home is an ongoing process that requires the use of many varied parameters and guidelines. Since assessment is the basis upon which quality care is planned and involves many factors, this entire chapter will focus on the types of information needed for the assessment process. The nurse will choose which parts of the assessment material to use on the basis of the needs of each specific patient, diagnosis, and situation. Although requirements for clinical expertise vary within organizations, the content of this chapter includes all information necessary for the home care nurse to use while assessing patients.

Health/Illness History

The assessment process should begin by using a health/illness history that involves both the verbal information given by the patient and the observations made during the visit. Home health nurses have the unique experience of observing the environment in which the patient lives and evaluating the effect of this environment on the patient's health and illness. Data gathered from taking the initial history can be used to determine the need to conduct a more in-depth assessment in various areas.

The assessment areas of medication, nutrition, mental status, activities of daily living, and family assessment have an important impact on planning care for patients in their homes. So that these areas can be more fully assessed, specific guidelines follow this section. The subjective information gathered through the comprehensive history-taking process can then be used to determine focus areas when conducting the physical assessment.

Everyone involved in home health care must see the value of spending adequate time in conducting a complete assessment. Only by taking the time necessary to fully assess the patient can the plan of care be developed accurately and can the care be directed to the real cause/effect of the problem. Missing the opportunity to assess the individual patient's situation thoroughly means a misdirected plan of care that results in a great deal of money wasted and a prolonged problem situation for the patient.

Content of the History

By definition, a health/illness history includes anything that will have bearing on the patient's current or future health status. The list below outlines the main areas included in a basic Health/Illness History. The areas marked with an asterisk indicate those specific assessment guidelines that follow in a separate section. These sections should be used when the patient situation indicates more information is needed relative to these areas.

1. Current Illness or Health Status

- When the problem started.
- Describe the course—is it improving or getting worse?
- The current status of the condition.
- What makes it better, what makes it worse?
- What prompted the patient to seek help, what does the patient think the problem is, and what help does the patient want?
- Current medications and diet and the patient's reaction (see page 100).
- Current treatments.

2. Past History

- Previous physical problems including surgery, accidents, major injuries, serious illnesses, and the dates when care was received.
- Previous emotional/mental problems with the dates and treatments.

- Preventive practices, that is, Pap smears, dentist, eye exams, and such.
- Allergies to food, medication, and environment.

3. Family History* (*See* page 47)

- Any predisposition to disease.
- Any recent physical problems in family members.

4. Personal and Social History

- Occupational history—type of employment, hazardous exposure.
- Educational background—check to see if patient can read by asking them to read their medication label.
- Religious practices—including church membership and clergy of choice.
- Cultural influences and language barriers—what is their primary language?
- Socioeconomic status—income sources, ability to meet basic needs, involvement with financial assistance organizations.
- Present concerns, outlook, self-esteem.* (*See* page 40)
- Relationships with family members and community.* (*See* page 47)

5. Safety Status* (*See* pages 107 to 111)

- Mobility
- Living arrangement
- Main caregiver
- Physical layout of home

6. Lifestyle Habits

- Use of alcohol, caffeine, tobacco, drugs
- Hobbies, recreation (type and frequency)
- Coping ability
- Pattern of exercise
- Sleep patterns
- Elimination habits

Assessment Items in a Psychological Exam

Previous History

Many medical illnesses present psychiatric symptoms. It is important to rule out any underlying physical problem before attributing the symptom to a psychiatric disorder. This step is especially true of symptoms that have a sudden onset. When there is a known history of a psychiatric disorder, information should be obtained about the following:

- Duration of the problem
- Frequency of symptoms
- Type of symptoms the patient is experiencing
- Current and past treatment and its result

Sensory Perceptions and Thinking

Disturbances in sensory perception include hallucinations, illusions, distortions of sensory experience, and some misinterpretations of sensory perceptions. Thinking disturbances include changes in rate of thinking, loose association, incoherence, flight of ideas, obsessions, compulsions, and delusions.

All of these symptoms are frequently associated with mental disorders. If there is evidence of alterations in sensory perceptions and/or thinking during the course of routine assessment, these alterations should be explored further. To assist in further assessing these altered states, the following definitions are given so assessment can be more differential.

Delirium   Since delirium can occur as a result of physical conditions, it is important to distinguish the symptoms of delirium from psychotic disorders and dementia. The following are diagnostic criteria used to identify delirium as a problem.

1. Clouding of consciousness—a reduced clarity of

awareness of environment, with reduced capacity to shift, focus, and sustain attention to environmental stimuli.
2. At least two of the following:

- Perceptual disturbance: misinterpretations, illusions, or hallucinations
- Speech that is at times incoherent
- Disturbance of sleep-wakefullness cycle with insomnia or daytime drowsiness
- Increase or decreased psychomotor activity

3. Disorientation and memory impairment.
4. Clinical features develop over a short period of time (usually hours to days) and tend to fluctuate over the course of the day.
5. Evidence, from the history, physical examination, or laboratory tests, of a specific organic factor judged to be etiologically related to the disturbance.

Hallucinations   Some types of hallucinations are more commonly associated with organic or toxic states than with emotional disorders. These hallucinations must be assessed as related to the physical condition and treated as such rather than mislabeled as a psychological condition. These types of hallucinations include:

- Visual Hallucinations: Simple patterns such as lines, dots, flashes of light; small insects; spiders; rodents; and miniature people.
- Auditory Hallucinations: simple sounds, bells, buzzing, and voices when in a clouded sensorium.
- Tactile Hallucinations: Insects crawling over the skin, infestation of body by insects and phantom limb pain.

Level of Consciousness

The level of consciousness (LOC) ranges from alert to comatose. When levels of consciousness are identified it is important to realize that most alterations in LOC are due to an underlying pathological physical problem, not a psychological one.

Depression

In the setting of acute or chronic illness, depression is frequently a concomitant condition. If asked point blank, patients will often relate that they feel depressed, down, blue, or more tearful than usual. Since it is important to measure behaviors instead of "labeling" people, depression should be suspected if the following symptoms are present:

1. Appetite disturbances (either weight gain or weight loss).
2. Lowered mood (varying from mild sadness to intense feelings of guilt and hopelessness).
3. Difficulty thinking.
4. Inability to concentrate or make decisions.
5. Loss of interest in work, recreation, or activity.
6. Somatic complaints (headache, sleep disturbances, insomnia or hyposomnia, decreased sexual drive).
7. Psychomotor retardation or agitation.
8. Suicidal ideation.

Cognitive Functioning and Memory Loss

Since a large percentage of elderly patients require services from home health agencies, home care nurses must deal with patients with impairments of cognitive functioning and memory loss every day. Either as a presenting problem or a secondary diagnosis, the severity of senile dementia can be assessed in the course of doing a routine admission assessment through the use of a simple mental status examination.

Assessing a patient's level of cognitive functioning is important to not only evaluate their current status, but to provide a baseline of information for use in the future. Some agencies and hospitals now require a mental status evaluation for all patients over the age of 65 upon each admission for service to provide this baseline.

Definition

Organic mental disorder is the current terminology used to describe mental disorders with a known cause related to structural damage, operational malfunction of the brain, or a known metabolic disturbance. Dementia is the most common organic mental disorder a home health nurse will encounter.

Dementia is a global decline of memory and cognitive functioning significantly below what is expected for a given individual based on previous performance, education, and achievement in the absence of altered consciousness. Dementia is a behavioral diagnosis.

While there are several types of dementia, the term senile dementia of the Alzheimer type (SDAT) is commonly used in professional literature.

Causes and Treatment

The primary cause of dementia is Alzheimer's disease. Other conditions that can cause dementia are: multiple infarcts (CVAs), Parkinsonism, Pick's disease, Huntington's disease, and Wilson's disease. For the most part, these conditions are not treatable.

Some causes of dementia are potentially treatable. These include dementia caused by drugs and alcohol, tumors, nutritional deficiencies, infections, metabolic imbalance, inflammatory disease, endocrine disorders, trauma, and psychiatric/neurologic conditions.

Mental Status Assessment

A simple mental status examination can be conducted during the routine admission assessment and subsequent visits by integrating questions in history taking, implementing interventions, and general discussion with the patient and family. The following areas will be helpful in organizing specific areas to be addressed. After this list of assessment areas, a formal mental status questionnaire which can be used to score individuals for diagnostic purposes, is found.

Orientation

Person Can they give you their name, name of relatives, physician, person to contact in an emergency? If so, they are oriented as to person.

Place   Ask them for their address and telephone number, also to show you around the house identifying rooms, locations of medications, phone, treatment supplies, and anything else that is essential to their ability to live in their residence. Most of the time, it is more important a person is able to navigate in their environment than to know their address.

Time   Ask date. If they don't know the date, progress in asking the day of the week, the month, the year, and lastly if they are unable to answer any of the previous items, ask them which season of the year it is. They are partially oriented if they miss one or more items.

Memory

Recent   Obtain history about recent events, for example, dates of hospitalization, reason for hospitalization, prescribed medication and treatments. You will need to verify if their answers are accurate based on the information you have.

Intermediate   Ask about past medical and social history. Again verification is important.

Remote   Ask their date of birth. Generate discussion about their past such as where they were born, how long they have lived in their community, when married, and any other significant events of the past you can verify.

If a person can give a fairly good, coherent medical history they most likely have little memory impairment. Evaluate more closely someone who confuses you as they present their history.

Judgement

Ask what they would do in an emergency. Is this appropriate? Have they demonstrated poor judgement in their own medical care, such as, failure to treat a problem or taking inappropriate treatments?

Appearance

Assess their personal hygiene. Are clothes appropriate for the weather? Is there a decline in hygiene? Ask family to verify their response if you have doubts as many patients will tend to deny any problems.

Activities of Daily Living

Is there a reported decline in the patient's ability to manage ADLs not related solely to a physical problem? Is the patient able to manage finances? Is there a decrease in participation in social activities or increase in irritability in a social situation? Is the patient beginning to refuse to go out shopping or visiting? These may be early signs of cognitive impairment and should be documented and observed for further deterioration. (See page 107 for more specific criteria.)

Abstraction

Thinking can be either abstract or concrete. The ability to think abstractly diminishes with cognitive impairment. When a person thinks concretely they have a difficult time understanding ideas and concepts. Teaching needs to be geared to this literal way of thinking. To test for abstraction ask someone similarities of various items or how to interpret proverbs. The nurse only needs to do this if the patient doesn't seem to understand teaching and the problem isn't due to memory loss.

Other Factors

Is there a reported change in the patient's ability to get around in the community? Does the patient loose items frequently? Is there a change in driving behavior such as erratic driving, very slow driving, traffic tickets, others reporting unsafe driving practices, or loss of car in parking lot?

Mental Status Questionnaire

The following questionnaire consists of 10 questions found to be valid and reliable indicators for measuring mental status of patients. These questions cover orientation for time, place, and person; memory—recent or remote; and general information or "intellectual capacity." The presumed mental status rating is described by using the term Chronic Brain Syndrome. As discussed earlier, organic mental disorder is the currently used terminology.

When administering the questionnaire, remember to have the patient's full attention and adjust your questions for any sensory disorder such as difficulty in hearing. You may either ask the questions directly as written in a formal way or integrate the questions in your conversation so as not to call attention to the fact that you are administering a questionnaire.

The rating of the test is listed on the chart. If a patient makes less than three errors on the questionnaire but appears to have poor memory or other intellectual difficulties, an affective disorder may be present, and a referral may be needed.

Mental Status Questionnaire (MSQ)

	Question	Presumed Test Area
1.	Where are we now?	Place
2.	Where is this place located?	Place
3.	What is today's date—day of the month?	Time
4.	What month is it?	Time
5.	What year is it?	Time
6.	How old are you?	Memory—recent or remote
7.	What is your birthday?	Memory—recent or remote
8.	What year were you born?	Memory—recent or remote
9.	Who is president of the U.S.?	General information—memory
10.	Who was president before him?	General information—memory

Rating of MSQ

Number of Errors	Presumed Mental Status
0–2	Chronic Brain Syndrome, absent or mild
3–5	Chronic Brain Syndrome, mild to moderate
6–8	Chronic Brain Syndrome, moderate to severe
9–10	Chronic Brain Syndrome, severe
Non-testable	Chronic Brain Syndrome, severe

NOTE: This questionnaire is modified from: Kahn, RL, Goldfarb, AI, Pollack, M, and Peck A, *American Journal of Psychiatry*, 1960, page 326.

Family Assessment

In addition to the Health/Illness History, you can learn much about the patient's situation by an assessment of the family. Viewing the patient within the context of the family can help to develop a clearer picture of the environment.

The environment affects not only the patient's illness but also how successful the interventions will be and how long they will take. Since most patients depend on family members or other caregivers to assist with their care while recovering from an illness, the role of the family is most important. Often patients have friends and neighbors who act as their family both in an emotional and supportive caregiver role. The following guidelines can be used to assess their interaction with the patient also.

Purpose

1. The home care nurse needs to know how to mobilize resources to cope with current illness and future plans.

By understanding how the family interacts, interventions can be more specific and effective.

2. Families are often not aware of how their system works, and raising it to their consciousness can help them accent the positives and perhaps look to change the negatives.

3. The family system in place may need to be revamped in view of the presenting problem so families can be helped with anticipatory guidance to avoid crisis situations. This fact is especially true in families learning to cope with a member's long-term chronic disease.

Process

Although many tools and formats for family assessment can be used to guide observations, it is important to rely on professional judgement through subjective data and observation to fully determine the family's ability to contribute to the plan of care. Following is an overview of the process of family assessment followed by guidelines to the assessment.

1. **Focus on the family, not the member.** Since the family is a unit itself, it is imperative the nurse observe the family separately from the assessment of its individual members.

2. **Allow adequate time for data collection**. The collection of data to form a valid family assessment takes time and is ongoing throughout the time the patient is on service. Do not make all decisions relative to this complex assessment after the first or second visit. Validate your impressions by asking family members if your observations are correct.

3. **Assessment can be quantitative as well as qualitative**. Some agencies have forms that are useful in rating the assessment of the family. Additionally, this type of measurement makes it easier to make referrals and judgements based on sound information that can be gradiated. Family assessment tools, however, should be used with care since this assessment is highly subjective and relies greatly on the knowledge base of the professional nurse.

4. **Emphasize family strengths**. Focus a great deal of attention on the strengths the family possesses and how these strengths can be used in the plan of care. Clarifying the strengths will be important as you develop the plan and contract outlined in Chapter 1.

Guidelines for Family Assessment

The guidelines that follow provide a framework for organizing information about the various families encountered in practice. Remember, in some families, questions may be of a more sophisticated level; in others, basic questions using simple language are necessary.

1. **Family constellation**—Each members name, occupation, and educational background.
2. **Economic status**—Are there adequate resources to meet basic life requirements?
3. **Role of individuals in family**—Are stereotypic roles followed or, if different constellation than nuclear family, what role do people assume? Is there flexibility of role definition such that family members can cover for each other in cases of illness?
4. **Communication patterns within the family**—Who talks to whom about what, and who is the leader/decision maker of the family.
5. **Significant change in family life**—Have there been major changes in recent past as well as the change brought about by the current problem?
6. **Coping ability of family**—How do they cope as a family? How does each individual cope?
7. **The energy level of the family**—Who takes on major responsibilities and tasks? What is the effect of that on the entire family?
8. **Decision-making process**—How are decisions made and by whom?
9. **Support systems**—What are the internal and external systems that give the family support? Some external systems may be church, work, associations, and clubs, some internal systems may be extended family members.
10. **History of use of health care**—How has the family reacted to health problems in the past, how do they

relate to their primary care providers, what plans do they have for emergencies, what health beliefs do they have? Are they willing and able to seek and accept assistance from outside sources?

Characteristics of a Healthy Family

1. There is a facilitative process of interaction among family members.
2. They enhance individual member development.
3. Role relationships are structured effectively.
4. They actively attempt to cope with problems.
5. They have a healthy home environment and lifestyle.
6. They establish regular links with the broader community.

Physical Assessment

When the information from the health/illness history, family assessment, and the general psychological assessment has been gathered, the physical assessment can then be conducted in an efficient manner. All patients will receive a physical assessment to the extent deemed necessary by the patient's condition, standards of practice used by the organization, ability of the nurse, and policies of the agency. The following guidelines for physical assessment may be used as a reference when completing this aspect of the assessment.

It is not the purpose of this section to replace the several excellent texts available to the home care nurse in learning and reviewing physical assessment. I suggest that a nursing agency have several texts (such as those listed in the references at the end of the book) available for nurses to consult between home visiting. This section is a brief outline that highlights those aspects of physical assessment which will be most commonly used by the nurse in home visiting. It is presented in a format concise enough for the nurse to consult while in the home.

When conducting a physical assessment in the home environment, always think of the areas that need to be covered as they relate to the patient situation. Although the following section is explicit, it is not meant to imply that all aspects should be conducted on all patients on every admission and visit. However, as the illness severity of patients seen in the home increases, it becomes increasingly important that the home care nurse be able to use professional expertise to determine which areas need to be assessed on each encounter with the patient.

Definition

Physical assessment is a deliberate, ordered process of examination whereby physical, objective evidence of disease is determined to be absent or, if present, quantified. Such assessment is accomplished by interviewing, inspection, palpation, percussion, auscultation, and mensuration.

Purpose

The purposes of a physical assessment in the home are:

- To establish baseline data against which future changes in the patient's condition can be evaluated. This is especially important since the in-depth data documented in the patient's hospital or physician office chart are not always available to the nurse in the home.
- To discover any infirmity that may not have been reported in the referral to the home health agency.
- To establish rapport with the patient. The process of eliciting the history and completing a physical examination assures the patient that the nurse knows his/her individual situation—a factor that can be instrumental in eliciting the patient's compliance with therapy.
- To monitor for changes in the patient's condition.
- To evaluate the effect of interventions.
- To assess the severity of problems which the patient may express concern about at the initial or subsequent visits.
- To collect and present information about the patient's condition that is thorough and organized, thereby giving the primary care provider better information upon which to base future decisions about patient care.

Equipment

The following equipment is necessary for the nurse to carry out the various aspects of physical assessment. It is up to the home health agency and the nurse to determine which supplies are essential and to provide those for home visiting.

1. **Stethoscope:** Each nurse should own a personal stethoscope so that the ear pieces fit properly. The tubing should not exceed 15 inches and the head should have both a bell and a diaphragm.
2. **Sphygmomanometer:** It should be recalibrated frequently with a regular size cuff. The agency should have a wide cuff available, as using too small a cuff will give an overestimation of the arterial pressure. The inflatable bladder should cover two-thirds the length of the upper arm, and reach one-half way around the arm to give the proper compression.
3. **Scale:** The agency should have accurate scales available for nurses to take on home visits for when patients do not have accurate equipment.
4. **Tape Measure:** Calibrated in centimeters.
5. **Tuning Fork:** For testing vibratory sense, a fork of 128 cycles per second is needed.
6. **Safety Pin:** Used for sensory testing.
7. **Thermometers:** Both rectal and oral.
8. **Urine Collection Cups.**
9. **Urine Testing Dipsticks:** Multiple tests are available on the dipsticks. As a minimum, glucose, pH, and blood sensitivity are needed.
10. **Stool Guiac Testing Equipment:** Cardboard slides and fresh developer. Note the expiration date, and recall that developer left open is not accurate.
11. **Otopthalomoscope:** These should be available for nurses to use.
12. **Tongue Blades.**
13. **Flashlight or Penlight:** A good source of light is not often available in the home.

Procedure

The following table outlines a head-to-toe progression of the physical examination. The *How* column indicates what and how to assess each body system, as practical for the nurse on a home visit. The *Normal* column indicates the range of normal findings. The *If Abnormal* column suggests appropriate actions for the more common causes of abnormal findings.

Head-to-Toe Progression of Physical Examination

How	Normal	If Abnormal
Vital Signs There should be an ongoing log documenting the patients vital signs. In any communication with the primary care provider these statistics should be reported.		
Weight and Height Some estimate of the patient's height should be recorded. The patient should be weighed on the initial visit. If the patient doesn't have a scale, the nurse should bring one.	*See Normal Weight/Height Table—Appendix A* Many adults are concerned about their weight. It is useful to compare the patient's height and weight to the standardized charts. Body weight more than 20% above the normal range has been demonstrated to pose a health risk.	An adult can accumulate 10 pounds of fluid before it will be detectable as pitting edema.

All patients should be weighed at least every 4–6 weeks. This timing should be increased for anyone with digestive complaints, on diuretics, any time dehydration is considered, and in the presence of any question about worsening cardiac status.

In encouraging weight reduction, it is generally more useful to set a goal based on the patient's desired weight as many obese adults have never been weighed within the normal range and consider such a goal impossible.

Explore the concept of obesity with patients who are underweight, as well, as some will be found to have a mistaken self concept of obesity and be dieting in spite of subnormal weight. This can have many clinical ramifications.

Blood Pressure

The patient's blood pressure (B/P) should be recorded every visit. If a different size cuff than normal is used, that should be noted. Which limb the pressure was taken on, the position the patient was in, and the pulse should be recorded with each B/P reading.

See Cardiovascular Assessment

(Continued)

Physical Examination—Continued

How	Normal	If Abnormal
Pulse The pulse rate should be recorded with an indication of whether the pulse is regular, irregularly irregular, or regularly irregular. If the pulse is irregular, count for a full minute. It is also useful to count apically if in doubt.	See Cardiovascular Assessment	If a previously regular pulse becomes irregular, other signs of worsening cardiac status should be assessed.
Respirations The respiratory rate should be counted initially and any time there is suspicion that the patient is in distress. Patients with respiratory diagnoses should have respiratory rate noted frequently.		If respiratory rate is increased, look for other indicators of distress or infection.
Temperature Record at initial visit and any time there is a suspicion of infection.	Normal range (oral): 97–99.6 °F 36.2 ° – 37.6 °C	

Oral temperature: Don't take within 15 minutes of ingesting food or liquid and wait at least 2 minutes after smoking. Accurate oral temperatures require that the thermometer remain in place for 8-9 minutes. More time may be required if the thermometer is coming in from storage in a cold car.

Temperature is lowest between 2 and 6 A.M. and highest between 4 and 7 P.M. because of the normal variation in cortisol levels which vary with the diurnal cycle.

The elderly do not always register a fever in response to infection. Other indicators of infection should, therefore, be assessed carefully.

Fever can signify many problems; infection and dehydration are two common problems.

Axillary temperature: The thermometer must be in place for 11 minutes for an accurate reading.

Axillary temperatures normally register slightly lower than oral temperatures.

Rectal temperature: The thermometer must be in place only 2-3 minutes for an accurate temperature.

Normal rectal temperatures are slightly higher than oral temperatures.

The patient must keep up fluid intake during a fever. If dehydration is the issue, you need to consider whether the dose of prescription drugs needs to be reduced to avoid overdosing.

(Continued)

Physical Examination—Continued

How	Normal	If Abnormal
Eyes		
Ask about recent changes in vision, any blurring, itching, or discharge	With increasing age it is more difficult to read fine print held close.	Refer
Test vision using a newspaper to assure that the patient can read regular size type, since this is used on prescriptions.	Using their prescriptive lenses, patients of all ages can normally see regular type. If unable to see regular type, try the headlines.	Be sure all instructions are written large enough for the patient to see. Large-print diet instructions are available.
	The line should appear straight, without any waviness, blurring, or any sections missing.	If the line ever appears distorted, the patient should be evaluated by an opthalmologist immediately.
Teach patients over 50 to test themselves for senile macular degeneration at least once a month: test each eye separately by looking at some straight line (a door trim or table leg for example).		
Recommend: Yearly eye exams for diabetics; glaucoma testing every 1-2 years for everyone over 40.		

Ears

Ask about decreased hearing on either side, any itching or discharge. Test hearing by placing a ticking watch against one ear, and then slowly move it away, having the patient indicate when the sound disappears. Compare with the opposite side.

Check to be sure that the distance the watch is from the ear is the same on both sides. This is a gross screening method that will not be accurate if there is background noise which is stronger on one side than the other.

With increasing age, the ability to hear high-pitch sounds decreases. It is useful to be certain one is speaking into an elders "best ear" and to intentionally speak in a lower pitch of voice.

An accumulation of cerumen is the most common cause for hearing loss. This is easily identified with an otoscope. If this is not found to be the cause, hearing testing is indicated.

Cerumen may be removed with a curette or preferably by irrigation with warm water directed at the walls of the canal from a 50-cc syringe. If the wax does not dislodge with irrigation, it can be softened by instilling mineral or olive oil 2-3 gtts. b.i.d. for 3-5 days, then repeat the warm water irrigation or instill hydrogen peroxide (H_2O_2) 2–3 times a day for two days.

Nose

Ask about discharge, bleeding, and ability to smell.

Increased discharge and bloody noses are commonly due to dry air.

Increase fluids and humidity.

(Continued)

Physical Examination—Continued

How	Normal	If Abnormal
To inspect the interior nose, have the patient hold head straight, then push the tip of the nose upward and shine the light straight in.	The mucosa of the nose is slightly more red than that of the mouth. Irritation from smoking makes it redder still. A bluish swollen mucosa is typical with allergies.	If decreased ability to smell, look for other cranial nerve deficits, and consider referral if patient troubled.
Check to see that both nostrils are patent, by occluding each separately and asking the patient to inhale.		A deviated septum is the most common reason for there to be a diminished air flow through one nostril. Surgery is required to correct this.
		If the occlusion is due to an infectious process, steaming can be helpful. Inhaling the steam from boiling water or hot vinegar may help. Decreasing the dryness by forcing fluids and a room humidifier may also be of use. Cold steamers are recommended. This problem espe-

cially occurs when people first start heating their houses in the fall. Encourage frequent cleaning of furnace and humidifier filters as they are a potential habitat for molds.

If there is any reason to suspect a foreign body, (unilateral, purulent discharge, or visualizing an unidentifiable object in a child), refer.

Any painful lesion should be referred. There is an increased risk of developing a cancer at any site where there is constant irritation, as from dentures rubbing.

These are cancer warning signals. If new and not previously evaluated, refer.

If there is an obvious droop, tactfully determine if the client has noticed it, and if so when it

(Continued)

A report of a painless state is not necessarily reassuring as serious lesions are often painless.

There should be none

Mouth and Throat

Ask about: Any pain or sores in the mouth. If they have dentures, do they rub anywhere. Any difficulty chewing food

Any difficulty swallowing or persistant hoarseness

Examine: General symmetry of the lips

Physical Examination—Continued

How	Normal	If Abnormal
		started. If it is new and has not been evaluated, it should be referred. Look for other evidence of neurologic deficits, especially the cranial nerves (See Neurologic Assessment, page 93).
The corners of the mouth for cracking	Neither side should appear to droop, although slight asymmetry is normal	If due to dryness, Vaseline at bedtime is useful (if the patient is not allergic to petroleum products). May suggest riboflavin deficiency, consider nutrition evaluation if persistent.
Gum line and teeth	Gum securely attached to teeth and clear of debris	Hypertrophy seen with dilantin therapy. Encourage thorough brushing b.i.d., flossing desirable every 24 hours; regular dental evaluations are recommended also.
Oral mucosa for lesions	Identify the parotid ducts on buccal mucosa at level of upper 2nd molars.	Any area of bleeding, white or velvety red lesions, or sores that don't heal should be re-

Throat for enlarged tonsils, post-nasal discharge, asymmetry	Identify sublingual salivary ducts to either side of frenulum. When patient says "ahhh," soft palate should raise symmetrically. Tonsillar tissue frequently atrophied or not visible in adults.	ferred. Persons who smoke and drink alcohol are especially at risk for head and neck cancer. Asymmetric soft palate in the absence of other neurologic findings should be mentioned to the physician at the next visit. If other neurologic symptoms are present, more immediate evaluation is suggested.
Neck Ask about stiffness or pain.	None	Pain and stiffness commonly due to tension manifest in the trapezius muscles.
Any sensation of fullness or pain in the thyroid area		Making slow deliberate circles with head can help to relax, as does neck massage and heat. Sleeping on too high a pillow can also cause neck pain. If due to arthritis or trauma, don't advise exercise. If positive, check for signs of thyroid disease.

(Continued)

Physical Examination—Continued

How	Normal	If Abnormal
Gently examine carotid pulses bilaterally	Symmetrical in strength (See scale for grading under cardiac exam)	May wish to mention to physician, especially if there is positive family history. Listen over artery with bell of stethoscope for bruit. If heard, it should be evaluated by a physician: nonemergent.
Examine lymph nodes: Occipital Pre- and Post-auricular Parotid Subramandibular Submental	No enlargement Group of nodes and area drained: Occipital: posterior scalp and deep neck Preauricular: forehead, upper face, and conjunctiva Postauricular: crown of scalp and part of ear Parotid: side of head, eye, ear, and nose Submandibular: chin, cheek, nose, teeth, tongue, and floor of mouth Submental: tongue and lower lip	If you find enlarged nodes, note location, size, number, tenderness, and mobility. Look for signs of infection in areas nodes drain. Supraclavicular nodes especially on the left are worrisome, as are hard, fixed, nontender nodes. Check for node enlargement elsewhere.

Cervical	Superficial cervical: skin and neck Deep cervical: larynx, thyroid, esophagus, and trachea	
Supra- and Infraclavicular	Supraclavicular: head, arm, chest wall, and breast Infraclavicular: axillary nodes and arm	
Lymph Nodes Ask if patient has noted any enlarged glands, or "lumps" in the neck, armpits, or groin.	Adults often have a few small "shotty" nodes in their groin from previous infections. These are small (<2cm), nontender, mobile nodes, and benign. Nodes may enlarge secondary to infection but should return to normal once infection resolved.	If patient has noted enlarged nodes, palpate them. If fixed, hard, nontender or if they persist, they should be evaluated. Record location, size, and number of nodes identified.
Examine by inspecting skin and palpating nodes in neck, as just discussed, and Axillary Lateral Pectoral Subscapular Central	Group of nodes and area drained: Lateral: drain arms, deltoid area, and anterior chest wall Pectoral: anterolateral chest wall, abdominal wall above umbilicus and breast Subscapular: Posterior chest wall and neck	

(Continued)

Physical Examination—Continued

How	Normal	If Abnormal
Epitrochlear Superior Inguinal Inferior Inguinal Popliteal	Central: Chest wall, breast, and arm Epitrochlear: Hand and forearm Superior Inguinal: Abdominal wall below umbilicus, buttocks and external genitalia Inferior Inguinal: leg and foot Popliteal: heel and lateral foot	
Breasts Ask about any masses, pain, discharge, dimpling, or other recent changes in men and women.	Fibrocystic breasts are normally bilaterally lumpy and may be tender premenstrually. Breast discharge may continue for 6 months after stopping breast-feeding.	
Ask about a family history of breast cancer.		If there has been breast cancer in a mother or sister, patient's risk is much greater, especially if that cancer developed premenopausally. Women with such a family history should be profes-

Examine each breast and axillary nodes by inspecting sitting, leaning forward, and laying down.

Palpate using pads of fingers, covering the entire breast tissue, including under the arm and under the nipple.

sionally examined at least yearly.

There should be no evidence of dimpling, both nipples should appear to point symmetrically.

Slight, generalized nodularity.

In large breasts, inframammary ridge often prominent (should be symmetrical).

Breast exams should be done just after menses.

Recent changes to asymmetry, newly developed inversion of one nipple, dimpling, swelling, redness, or discharge should be referred.

Most cancers occur in upper outer quadrant. Findings of masses that are firm, nontender and fixed are most worrisome. Any mass that stands out as different to the patient and/or to the examiner should be referred, as should any area of tenderness, even if no mass is felt. These findings generate so much anxiety that it is useful for the nurse to intervene to secure an early appointment for evaluation.

Reassurance that most masses are not serious can be helpful to the patient.

(Continued)

Physical Examination—Continued

How	Normal	If Abnormal
Recommend: Monthly self breast exams after menses or on first of month if menopausal. The American Cancer Society mammogram recommendations: every 2 years from 40-50, and yearly if over 50 for all women. If high risk, women should begin mammograms at 35. **Lungs/Thorax** Ask about any chest pain with breathing.		Common causes for pain with breathing are rib or muscle injury, pleuritic inflammation, or lung involvement. Attempt to reproduce the pain by pressing on the area where the pain is worst. Auscultate the area carefully. Report findings if significant.

Any cough, and if present, is it productive?	Early morning coughing is common with smokers and with postnasal drip. Coughing in the middle of the night can occur when the excess fluids collected in congestive heart failure shift to the lungs while recumbent.	A new cough is most worrisome if in the presence of any signs of infection or changing cardiac status. Report significant findings. A chronic cough needs to be evaluated as it is a cancer danger signal. If the cough is due to chronic bronchitis, the patient should be watched carefully for signs of infection. Look for any signs of worsening cardiac status. Quantify how much exertion it takes to become short of breath and record this to use as a measure against which to judge future improvement or deterioration.
Any difficulty breathing, and if so, what brings it on. Is the difficulty more on breathing in, out, or is it equal throughout the respiratory cycle?	Persons who have not been getting regular exercise often complain of shortness of breath on exertion, which occurs simply because they are physically out of shape. Asthmatics commonly experience difficulty exhaling.	
Check respiratory rate	Adults: 12–16 breaths/minute. Anxiety can increase rate.	
Examine the thorax by looking at the shape and for the normal curves of the spine. The patient needs to be standing to fully appreciate scoliosis.	The thorax should be symmetrical from side to side. The lateral measurement is, normally, roughly twice the front to back diameter in adults. Children and the elderly are normally	An increased front-to-back diameter is seen with chronic obstructive pulmonary disease (COPD). One can expect breath sounds to be distant with a "barrel chest."

(Continued)

Physical Examination—Continued

How	Normal	If Abnormal
	more "barrel chested." Normal aging also tends to cause the spine to be more kyphotic, but there should be no scoliosis.	Scoliosis is not treated after adolescence, but is often seen in the elderly.
Palpate the spinous processes for any tenderness.	No pain should be elicited.	Patients who have lost bone mass may feel tenderness, for example, women with osteoporosis or patients on steroids long term. If the finding is new it should be reported. If chronic, the spine should be regarded as fragile, hence any falls are especially dangerous and ROM of the neck should not be encouraged.
Examine the lungs for symmetry of expansion by standing behind the patient, placing your fingers around the patient's chest at the bra level with thumbs at the spine. Have the patient inhale deeply and look		Any obstruction in the airways can keep one lung or lung lobe from filling fully. A large accumulation of fluid can do likewise. Such a finding should be recorded in a baseline exam. If not previously present, look for

to see that your thumbs are both moved equidistance from the spine. This tells you that both lungs are inflating equally. Listen to air movement in the lungs, using the diaphragm of the stethoscope. Begin above the scapula on the patient's back and compare sounds by listening in symmetrical areas left and right. The patient should be instructed to breath with mouth open and to take slightly deeper than normal breaths. Cover the entire back, underarm, and anterior chest. Pay particular attention to the area under the right breast, as this is the only access to the right middle lobe.

Between upper scapula and to either side of upper sternum you hear ***Bronchial Breath Sounds***. Inspiration and expiration are about equal in length and quite loud. Sounds should be symmetrical except between upper scapula. The right main stem bronchus lies slightly more posterior than the left. Consequently the bronchial breath sounds may normally be somewhat louder on the right than the left in this area.

Over the rest of the lungs you hear ***Vesicular Breath Sounds***: Inspiration is heard as longer than expiration. The sounds are softer and more difficult to hear but should be symmetrical from one side to the other. Heart

other respiratory symptoms and report to physician.

Asymmetry: anything that selectively interferes with the movement of air can decrease breath sounds on the side affected. If sounds seem softer on one side, have the patient whisper "99" and again listen to the two sides, comparing for symmetry. To further test, ask the patient to say "99" while you listen right and left to compare if the sound is transmitted symmetrically.

These two extra tests help to corroborate the suspicion aroused by subtle changes in breath sounds. Such asymmetry should be recorded in a baseline assessment. If it is new, look for other signs and symptoms of abnormal cardiac and/

(Continued)

Physical Examination—Continued

How	Normal	If Abnormal
	sounds override hearing breath sounds on the left anteriorly. Anything that increases the distance between the stethoscope and the air movement in the lungs will make the sounds less audible, for example, a "barrel chest" or obesity.	or respiratory function and report.
		Extra sounds:
		Rales: Heard at the end of inspiration. They sound like the ripping of Velcro; "crackles." Generally heard at the lung bases. If heard, ask the patient to cough, and then listen to see if the rales are still present. If gone, note that rales clear with cough. Teach the patient to deep breath and cough 2-4 times a day to clear the normal secretions that form in the lungs. Rales result from air moving through an accumulation of secretions and into previously collapsed alveoli.
	Extra sounds can be produced by secretions that have accumulated high in the bronchial tree. This commonly occurs with an upper respiratory infection and gives rise to sounds that are heard either in inspiration, expiration, or both and are heard throughout both lung fields. Having the patient cough, and preferably clear the secretions, will cause the sounds to disappear. The presence of such	Patients with chronic lung disease

sounds on auscultation does not indicate lung involvement but rather just secretion accumulation in the upper airways.

may have a few rales chronically present in their lungs that will not clear with coughing. Record in the baseline assessment where on the chest the rales were heard and how far up from the lung bases the rales continue.

If a patient develops new rales, look for signs of infection, deterioration in cardiac or respiratory function, and report.

Wheezes: Musical sounds usually heard in expiration, but may be inspiratory as well. Indicate a narrowed airway. When severe, can be heard without a stethoscope.

Wheezing in an asthmatic indicates a need for emergent evaluation by primary care provider. Check for signs of infection or respiratory compromise (fast, shallow breathing, cyanosis, and obvious distress).

(Continued)

Physical Examination—Continued

How	Normal	If Abnormal
		In an asymptomatic individual, the presence of a persistent, isolated wheeze should be reported as it can result from a lesion pressing on an airway.
		Pleural Friction Rubs: A harsh rubbing sound that occurs with inspiration and expiration and sound close to the stethoscope. Caused by inflammation between the two layers of pleura, may be accompanied by pain with breathing. Note where on chest the rub is heard. Look for signs of infection and notify care provider.
Cardiovascular Ask about arrhythmias: sensation of the heart beating fast, irregular, or unusually hard.		New onset of any cardiac symptoms should be reported.

Ask about chest pain: angina has many forms besides the typical left chest pain radiating down left arm or up into jaw. Any chest discomfort precipitated by exertion should raise suspicion. Be especially attentive to any such complaints in persons with history of cardiac disease, hypertension, and diabetics having previous "heart attacks."

If the patient is having chest pain chronically, record how much exertion it takes to cause it and/or how many nitroglycerine are needed per week, or day and per episode.

This serves as a baseline for future comparison. Increasing frequency or severity of angina should be reported as it indicates increasing compromise.

Ask about known heart disease: murmurs, congestive heart failure, previous admissions for heart problems.

It is helpful to know if the patient recalls that they have a murmur, although a negative response doesn't assure one that no murmur is present.

Ask about arteriolar disease: None
1) Angina (as earlier); 2) claudication: pain occurring in the calves or buttocks with exertion;

Check for symmetry of dorsalis pedis and posterior tibial pulses

(Continued)

Physical Examination—Continued

How	Normal	If Abnormal
3) unusually cold extremities; 4) hypertension. Ask about venous disease: Varicose veins, ankle swelling, phlebitis, or history of blood clots in the legs or in the lungs.	None Slight ankle swelling is normal at the end of the day when the patient has been on his/her feet, especially in hot weather. It is also commonly seen after prolonged sitting with feet dependent, especially in the elderly.	With the patient standing, inspect the posterior calves for varicose veins (see Examination of the Veins).
Examine the peripheral vascular system: Arteries: Inspect the extremities for any signs of decreased perfusion: asymmetric temperature or loss of hair on the dorsum of the digits, accompanied with diminished or absent pulse.	Hair distribution and temperature should be symmetrical between the two hands and the two feet.	Arterial insufficiency produces a cool, pale extremity with shiny atrophic skin and hair loss. The lack of oxygen to these tissues may cause pain and a spontaneous ulcer to occur. The tissue is especially susceptible to trauma and will be slow to impossible to heal.
Palpate all pulses: Temporal Carotid	Normal pulse rate in adults: 60-100 beats/minute (Persons who do regular vigorous aerobic ex-	If the pulse seems diminished on one side, listen over that pulse point with the bell of the steth-

Brachial
Radial
Femoral
Popliteal
Dorsalis Pedis
Posterior Tibial
Use the fingertips of both hands and check the right and left pulse at the same time, assessing for symmetry.

Pulses may be graded:
Absent = 0
Markedly diminished = 1
Moderately diminished = 2
Slightly diminished = 3
Symmetrical = 4
Using the proper size cuff the B/P should be taken on bare upper arm.

Record the onset of sounds and the cessation of sounds.

Record which position the patient was in and from which limb the pressure was taken.

ercise may normally have a lower heart rate)
Bradycardia: <60 beats/minute
Tachycardia: >100 beats/minute
The pulse should be regular, which can include a slight speeding of the pulse during inspiration.
For the most accurate measure, count the rate at the apex of the heart using the diaphragm of the stethoscope

Normal blood pressure in an adult is 140/90.

There can be a difference of 5–10 mm Hg in the reading between arms normally.

oscope for a bruit. This finding corroborates diminished flow, though is not always heard.

If the pulse is irregular, determine if it is regularly irregular or irregularly irregular. This provides a baseline for comparison on future examinations.

High blood pressure:
Recheck B/P on two or more occasions.
If over 140/90 the patient should be under supervision.

(Continued)

Physical Examination—Continued

How	Normal	If Abnormal
	In the asymptomatic person, the lower the blood pressure, the lower the risk of end organ damage.	Persons who are getting too much antihypertensive medication, are volume depleted (dehydrated or bleeding), have been on prolonged bedrest, or have compromised function of the autonomic nervous system. Diabetics are an example of the latter.
		Hypotension is experienced by the patient as dizziness or feeling of fainting upon standing.
If any of the readings needs to be rechecked, deflate the cuff fully and wait 2-3 minutes for normal circulation to resume before taking another reading.	Elderly persons are at greater risk for orthostatic hypotension.	
Patients on antihypertensive drugs should be checked lying, sitting and standing frequently. The pulse rate should be taken and recorded likewise.	Normally when a patient goes from lying to sitting or standing, the systolic blood pressure will drop only slightly, or it may stay the same.	If the blood pressure drops more than 10 mm Hgs and the pulse rate increases, ask the patient about symptoms of dizziness or lightheadedness. If present, there is a greater risk of falling. Such findings should be reported, and the patient cau-

tioned to arise by first sitting on the edge of the bed and then standing, and hold on to something for a minute before attempting to walk.

If varicosities are present, the patient is much more susceptible to forming clots.

Prolonged bedrest or periods with the feet dependent are especially worrisome. Under such conditions, the legs should be examined regularly for any signs of tenderness, cords or redness. To check for deep venous phlebitis, squeeze the back of the calf forward against the tibia. When possible, compare the two legs. Any increased tenderness on one side should be reported.

(Continued)

None

Examine the Veins

Inspect feet and legs for varicose veins. With the patient standing, look for enlarged tortuous vein on the calves, behind the knees, and onto the thighs. The large "ropey" looking veins indicate involvement of the deep venous system and are more worrisome than the fine superficial veins that patients complain about.

Physical Examination—Continued

How	Normal	If Abnormal
Check for Edema Press the soft tissues against the bone on the dorsum of the foot, behind the medial malleolus, and over the shin. If present, record: 1. How high up the shin the edema is present. 2. Grade the degree by estimating the depth of the pit in millimeters. 3. Chronic severe edema can be monitored by measuring the girth of the calf at a specified distance above the medial malleolus. Such measurement gives precise data to use as a baseline, hence, it is preferred over the subjective system of grading edema as "two plus." Bedridden patients accumulate edema over the sacrum. Check for this by pressing the soft tis-	None	Edema of one leg suggests impaired venous return of that leg. Bilateral edema may be due to bilateral venous insufficiency, having both legs dependent, impaired lymphatic drainage, or congestive heart failure (CHF). Chronic venous insufficiency and edema results in the skin becoming thickened and brown and can eventuate in ulcers at the ankle. Swelling of acute onset should be reported. In monitoring chronic conditions quantifying the de-

sue over the bones in the sacral area the same as in the legs. Note how high it ascends up the back and sides.		gree of abnormality is important, that is, the exact size of stasis ulcers, or amount of edema.
Examine the Heart		
Inspect the chest wall overlying the heart for symmetry and any visible pulsations.	Chest should look symmetrical. The point of maximal impulse (PMI) may be visible in the left 5th intercostal space. The PMI is generally caused by the motion of the apex of the heart.	The PMI is displaced laterally with left ventricular hypertrophy and in late pregnancy.
Palpate the aortic, pulmonic, tricuspid, and mitral areas for thrills (a sensation like the purring of a cat, caused by increased turbulence). Use the palm of the hand.	None	Record this finding for future comparison, though this will not generally change acutely. If a thrill is felt one can expect to hear a loud murmur since the blood flow is so turbulent.
Palpate for a sternal heave by placing the heel of your right hand over the lower end of the sternum.	None	If the sternum lifts with each heart beat there is right ventricular hypertrophy.
Auscultate the heart with the patient supine. Listen to all four valvular areas with the dia-	The pulsation of the abdominal aorta is observable between the sternum and umbilicus normally. Diaphragm best for high-pitched sounds Bell best for low-pitched sounds	

(continued)

Physical Examination—Continued

How	Normal	If Abnormal
phragm and then the bell of the stethoscope.		
Note the rate and rythym (regular, regularly irregular, or irregularly irregular)	See description of rate under pulses.	Record in baseline assessment for future comparison.
		If a heart rhythm converts from regular to irregular it should be reported.
Presence and comparison of S_1 and S_2 amplitude	S_1 is loudest at the apex (bottom) of the heart. It is caused by the closure of the mitral and tricuspid valves. S_2 is loudest at the base (top) of the heart. It is caused by the closure of the aortic and pulmonic valves.	
Splitting of sounds: Are S_1 and S_2 each single sounds, or are either or both of the sounds split into two audible components?	Physiological splitting: It is normal to hear a split of S_2 with inspiration in the pulmonic area. The time between S_1 and S_2 is	

systole. The time between S_2 and the next S_1 is diastole.

Systolic murmurs are common normally in children and may be heard in pregnancy, anemia, and fever. Systolic murmurs, thus may not indicate serious heart disease, but diastolic murmurs are always worrisome.

Murmurs:
Heard as a longer sound; a swishing, caused by extra turbulence of blood moving through the heart valves. If heard, record:
1. Where on chest wall heard the loudest
2. Whether it radiates and where to
3. Whether it is systolic or diastolic (systolic murmurs coincide with carotid pulse)
4. Whether high pitched or low pitched (high-pitched murmurs heard best with diaphragm, low-pitched murmurs heard best with bell)
5. Rate the loudness:
I/VI = very faint, not heard with every beat
II/VI = faint
III/VI = moderately loud
IV/VI = loud

Record the presence of a murmur and its characteristics in the baseline assessment.

Reassess it periodically to look for signs of worsening cardiac status.

(Continued)

Physical Examination—Continued

How	Normal	If Abnormal
V/VI = loud and accompanied with thrill VI/VI = can be heard with stethoscope off chest, accompanied with thrill.		
Extra Heart Sounds: *Systolic clicks* Clicks are differentiated from split sounds by their difference in pitch when compared with the heart sounds. The sound is a brisk click.	None	If there is a new sound heard that was not present at the time of the baseline assessment, look for signs of worsening cardiac status and report.
Early systolic clicks: Heard right after S_1 and are caused by the opening of aortic or pulmonic valve.		
Mid-to-late systolic clicks associated with the mitral valve.		

Diastolic Extra Sounds:

S_3: Heard right after S_2. Sound made by blood entering the ventricles. Heard best with the bell at the heart apex with the patient in the left lateral decubitus position.

Normal in persons under 40 In older persons it is heard when there is heart failure. Causes a characteristic "gallop" rhythm.

This sound appears acutely with decompensating congestive heart failure. Listen for it in patients with symptoms or history of such disease.

S_4: Heard right before S_1. Sound made when atrial contraction forces blood into ventricles that have increased resistance. Heard best with the bell and most commonly at the apex.

Many older persons will have an S_4 without other signs of cardiac disease.

Record in baseline assessment, as is useful to know about before attempting to evaluate the onset of new pathology.

Opening snap: Heard right after S_1. Sound made by the opening of a stenosed mitral valve. Heard best with the diaphragm along the lower heart border, it is a high-pitched, snapping sound.

None

Friction rub: A sound heard across both systole and diastole, caused by inflammation of the pericardial sac. Loud and heard across entire precordium.

None

Report immediately.

(Continued)

Physical Examination—Continued

How	Normal	If Abnormal
Abdomen Ask about the entire sequence of digesting food: Appetite: increase or decrease Nausea: any particular time of day or other precipitant Vomiting: relationship to meals Food intolerances: spices or fats	Gas-forming foods include the cabbage family, beans, roughage.	Chronic complaints about digestion should prompt the nurse to record weight frequently and check to see if symptoms could be due to medications. Refer acute symptoms
Pain: Onset, location, quality, ever had before, what makes better or worse, severity Gas: Increased belching or flatus Bowel Pattern: frequency, consistency, color; and specifically ask about tarry or blood stools, and recent changes in bowel habits.	Blood, if accompanied by pain, may just be from hemorrhoids but should be referred.	Change in pattern and/or blood are cancer danger signals.
Liver or Gallbladder disease		
Abdominal surgeries: sequellae Urination: burning, frequency,	Adults need 8 glasses of fluid a	An enlarged prostate increases the

hesitation or urgency, recent onset of nocturia. Any blood or discharge. Incontinence.	day and should urinate every 2-3 hours when awake.	risk of urinary infections. Men with hesitancy should be asked frequently about burning with urination.
	Men often experience hesitancy in starting urine flow because of benign prostatic hypertrophy that comes with aging.	Cystitis is a frequent cause for incontinence.
	Stress incontinence is frequently a problem for post-menopausal women because of decreased estrogen and/or pelvic support. Medications and exercises can be helpful; patient needs a referral.	
Inspect the abdomen: Contour and symmetry	Rounded, distended, or flat.	Scaphoid if emaciated. Fluid accumulates laterally.
Skin Changes	Old straie are silver.	New straie are red to blue and indicate recent expansion in girth, as in ascites, acute weight gain, or pregnancy.
Visible Movement	Pulsations of the abdominal aorta are normally visible above the umbilicus, especially in thin individuals.	Suspect aneurism if the area of pulsation is >4 cm and pulses laterally rather than anteriorally.

(Continued)

Physical Examination—Continued

How	Normal	If Abnormal
Masses	Stool in the large intestine is at times palpable. If mass is stool it will not be present if rechecked on subsequent days.	With patient standing look for hernias in inguinal area, at the umbilicus, or at old surgical incisions.
		If mass is found determine size, location, is it tender, pulsatile, mobile. Possible etiologies include flatus, feces, fetus, fluid, fat, or fatal growth; also distended bladder.
		Periods of silence followed by high-pitched sounds and cramping suggest obstruction.
Auscultate in all four quadrants with diaphragm of stethoscope for small bowel sounds (before doing any palpating)	To determine that there are no sounds, you need to listen for at least 5 minutes and hear nothing. Normal bowel sounds vary depending on time of last meal relevant to examination.	
Palpate superficially using one hand lightly to feel for superficial masses. Cover entire abdomen, including	Irregularities in adipose tissue can commonly be felt diffusely and superficially.	

the super pubic area and inguinal lymph nodes. Repeat this process using a deeper, two-handed palpation to feel for any deep masses. Palpate for the liver edge and the spleen. Percussion is useful to identify the liver margin and to note any areas of dullness in the abdomen. Blunt percussion is used to test for liver and kidney (costovertebral angle; CVA) tenderness.

The normal spleen is not palpable.

The normal liver edge is smooth and nontender.

Liver dullness is normally 6-12 cm in the right midclavicular line, generally from the 5th interspace to the costal margin.

CVA tenderness that is asymmetrical suggests kidney infection. Check for temperature and for cystitis symptoms.

Rectal Examination

With patient in left lateral knee chest position, inspect from perineum to the sacrococcygeal area for asymmetry or excoriation.

Inspect anus for fissures and hemorrhoids

Skin in this area is normally more deeply pigmented.

Any open lesions, fissures, or masses should be carefully evaluated and discussed with the patients primary care provider.

Insert gloved and lubricated index finger into anus, directing finger tip in direction of umbilicus.

The normal prostate is 4 cms in length and projects less than 1 cm into the rectum. The edges of the gland should be readily identifiable. The gland nor-

If the prostate is hot or the patient complains of exquisite tenderness, avoid any palpation and refer.

(Continued)

Physical Examination—Continued

How	Normal	If Abnormal
Identify sacral prominence through posterior wall and use this as a landmark to assure palpating the entire circumference of the rectal wall. Feel for any masses. In the male, identify the prostate on the anterior wall, compare the two lateral lobes for tenderness, asymmetric firmness, and any masses. Estimate the size of the prostate.	mally enlarges with age but should still feel rubbery, non-tender, and without any masses.	Since only the posterior aspect of the gland is palpable, it is not always possible to determine the degree of enlargement by examination. The subjective data from the patient is more significant than the objective data gathered from examination.
Test stool for blood.	False positives can result from a diet of rare beef or pork, vitamin C, horseradish or aspirin. The physician may wish to have the patient avoid such foods for 48 hours and then collect samples from 3 consecutive stools for retesting.	Consult regular care provider.

Neuro/Musculoskeletal

Observe general habitus:
Level of consciousness
Mood, affect, appearance
Any obvious asymmetry, tics,
  tremors, paresis or atrophy
Swollen joints
Posture
Communication:
Able to receive message
Able to send message (speech au-
  dible, clear, organized and co-
  herent)
Gait
Use of Assistive Devices

In benign familial tremors you see
fine tremors of head, neck and/
or arms. When arms are out-
stretched you see fine flexion
extension of fingers.
Etiology = familial, anxiety,
caffeine, drugs, or hypogly-
cemia. Slight hyphosis is normal with aging.

Elderly normally process information more slowly.

Resting tremor typical of Parkin-
sons.

Intention tremor increases as
hand nears another object.
Makes performing fine skills
impossible.

Receptive aphasia: When cannot
understand the message.
Expressive aphasia: Understands
but cannot respond with words.
Dysarthria: Difficulty forming the
words because of a lack of precise control of muscles of phonation.

Cerebral Function (*See Mental Status
Assessment*, page 43):
In the process of history taking,
determine that person is oriented to person, place, and
time.

If there are questions about a persons mental status, the opinion
of a "most supportive other"
must be elicited.
Be sure that a normal mental status examination is recorded as
a baseline for future comparison.

If the person seems at all confused or disoriented, a detailed
mental status exam should be
done. (See Psychological Assessment, page 40).

(Continued)

Physical Examination—Continued

How	Normal	If Abnormal
Ask about: Muscular problems: weakness, stiffness, inability to perform any specific tasks like climbing stairs, getting up out of easy chair, or combing hair. Skeletal problems: stiffness or joint pain, sense of grating in a joint with range of motion. Symptoms at the site of an old fracture or sprain. Nerve Problems: Cranial Nerves: any difficulty with movement or sensation to face. Changes in ability to taste or smell. Peripheral Nerves: Any numbness, burning or tingling to extremities Cerebellum: difficulty performing fine motor tasks (handwork or turning screws). Difficulty		
	Elderly often note a decrease sense of taste.	
	A combination of deficits to sensory input can make the elderly especially prone to falls: cata-	Caution to sit at bedside for a few moments before attempting to stand, then to stand and hold

keeping balance when walking; "uncoordinated."	racts can interrupt visual orientation, and callouses and peripheral neuropathies can diminish feeling on the soles of the feet. The elderly are also more prone to orthostatic hypotension.	onto something for a good minute before attempting to walk. Elderly are especially at risk if taking antihypertensive medication in situations where the light is suddenly bright or is dim, after changing glasses or having eye surgery.
Cerebrum: Does the patient note any change in ability to remember or to concentrate? Difficulty following a movie or TV show, following a recipe or craft instructions.	Elderly normally may forget small details like why they went to the cupboard or where they left the keys. This needs to be differentiated from major memory deficits like getting lost in neighborhood or not paying bills.	If report significant change, complete mental status exam should be done. Acute changes are most worrisome.
Inspect the patient's movement ability: model and ask patient to follow: Raise forehead Close eyes tight Look up, down, and side to side Show teeth Stick out tongue Bite down hard Test vision	Observe for symmetry Cranial nerve 7 Cranial nerves 3, 4, and 6 Cranial nerve 7 Cranial nerve 12 Cranial nerve 5 Cranial nerve 2	If any deficits of cranial nerves are noted, check visual fields by testing each eye individually to ascertain that each can see in a full circle. This can be very important clinically.

(Continued)

Physical Examination—Continued

How	Normal	If Abnormal
Test hearing	Cranial nerve 8	Palpate joint for crepitus or increased heat. If acute, refer.
Test to see soft palate raises symmetrically	Cranial nerve 9 and 10	
Test general range of motion (ROM) and strength by having patient turn head side to side; forward and back, and shrug shoulders up.	Inspect joints for enlargement or redness as patient completes ROM. Cranial nerve 8	If there is limited ROM, determine if it is due to: pain; bone or joint dysfunction; muscle weakness; nerve dysfunction.
Make a circle with shoulder joints Hold arms out straight, then in sequence bend fingers, thumbs, wrists, elbows, and bring elbows up above ears.	Criteria for grading muscle strength: Normal: Complete ROM against gravity and resistance Good: Complete ROM against gravity and some resistance (that is, some diminished strength) Fair: Complete ROM against gravity Poor: Complete ROM if gravity eliminated (that is, passive ROM)	
Test hand strength by having patient squeeze your fingers.		

While Standing

Test range of motion of spine by twisting side to side, bending backward, and forward.

Test range of motion of legs by accomplishing a deep knee bend or by alternately flexing toes, ankle, knee, and hip of one leg, and then fully extending it. Repeat with other leg.

Test cerebellar function by having the patient stand with feet touching and, if accomplished, then close eyes and stand for 30 seconds without holding onto anything and without losing balance. Be certain to stand nearby so as to catch the patient should they start to sway. Cerebellar function may be further tested by having the person "walk the line"—walk heel to toe.

Test peripheral sensation:

Trace: evidence of muscle contracting but no joint movement
Zero: no evidence of muscle contraction

Ambulatory elderly can generally accomplish a deep knee bend, but for safety, hold their hands if they wish to attempt it.

This is the Romberg test. There should be no decrease in this ability with aging.

If cannot maintain balance with eyes shut, person is relying on visual stimuli to maintain orientation rather than normal proprioception. Use a cane may be indicated to prevent future falls.

(Continued)

Physical Examination—Continued

How	Normal	If Abnormal
Use 128 cps tuning fork, vibrating and held by the stem. Touch to the most distal joint of each great toe and midfinger, and at each joint ask the patient to indicate (with eyes closed) whether the fork is vibrating ("buzzing") or holding still. If patient cannot sense vibration, move up one joint at a time and finally inch up shin until vibration can be sensed. Record extent of numbness. If vibratory sense is gone, check sharp/dull, light touch, and finally position sense ("which way am I pointing your toe, toward or away from your nose?")	May be slightly decreased sensation with aging.	Diabetes and chronic alcohol use each can result in a numbness in the same distribution as wearing stockings and gloves. Vibratory sense is often the first to be lost. Patients with decreased sensory ability need to be informed of their loss and cautioned that they will not be able to sense injurious objects or temperature extremes so they are at increased risk for injury. They may also have more difficulty maintaining their balance as they cannot easily perceive when their feet are touching the floor or steps.
Test deep tendon reflexes (DTRs). The muscle must be relaxed, and the tendon must be slightly stretched.	Response should be symmetrical.	

Reflex	Cord level tested	Normal response	Grading reflex response
Brachioradialis	Cervical 5-6	elbow flexion, forearm supination	Grade 0 = Absent
Biceps	Cervical 5-6	elbow flexion	Grade 1 = Present but diminished
Triceps	Cervical 7-8	elbow extension	Grade 2 = Normal
Patellar	Lumbar 2-4	knee extension	Grade 3 = Brisk
Achilles	Lumbar 5-Sacral 2	plantar flexion of foot	Grade 4 = Hyperactive, often with clonus
			DTR response should be recorded in the baseline assessment. Acute changes in response grade or to asymmetry should cause clinician to seek other signs of deteriorating neurological status.

Skin, Hair, and Nails

Skin:
Ask about general increase in dryness. If scaling, is it generalized or patchy.

Skin is normally more dry during periods when homes are heated and also with aging.
Hair and nails also more prone to being dry and brittle with age.

Applying a lotion or cream immediately after showering serves to capture moisture and correct dry skin. Hot baths should be avoided. Bathing less frequently may be indicated.

(Continued)

Physical Examination—Continued

How	Normal	If Abnormal
Changes in Pigmentation Lesions: See Appendix B. Any changes in a wart or mole Any sores that do not heal Any unexplained bleeding Any masses or thickening	The range of normal is broad, and a full description is more than can be covered here. Ask about changes, examine and look up any lesion in question (see Appendix B). Definitive diagnosis often requires biopsy; only an extremely experienced examiner can determine when biopsy is indicated.	Yellow sclera = jaundice Yellow palms = carotene excess Depigmented areas can be due to topical fungal infection or to systemic diseases. Any changes in warts or moles should be referred, as should any lesions that do not heal or bleed spontaneously.
Bruising	The skin and vessels are more fragile in old age, hence, they will bruise with less trauma. The spontaneous development of larger ecchymosis should cause one to question more severe trauma, or a bleeding disorder.	Malignant melanoma is characterized by moles that have an irregular border, are multicolored, that is, red, white, and blue, mixed in with the brown and black. Any suspicious lesion should be referred.

Hair: Changes in texture Changes in distribution	Hair thins and becomes finer with advancing age. Men and women alike can experience balding at the temples and crown. The typical female pubic hair distribution is triangular; male pubic hair is more diamond shaped	Hair can become finer with hyperthyroidism. Asymmetry of hair distribution on the dorsum of fingers or toes can be indicative of diminished arterial blood flow
Nails: Ask about changes in texture	With aging, nails become more brittle, thicken and may have a more yellow hue (especially toenails)	Many systemic conditions are reflected in the nails. (Consult bibliography for some assessment references.)
Inspect skin, hair and nails for color, texture, lesions, abnormal growth	Record specific description in baseline assessments.	
Inspect nail beds for clubbing and rapidity of capillary refill	Looking across the nail there should be a 160° angle between the base of the fingernail and the finger. The nail should feel firm against the nailbed.	Clubbing indicates some form of cardiorespiratory disorder. It is a non-specific sign.

Medication and Nutritional Assessment

Since concerns about medication and nutrition take up a great deal of a home care nurse's time, it is extremely important that an in-depth assessment be done on these two areas as part of the Health/Illness History. Basic assessment in these two areas needs to be thorough so that accurate plans are developed and baseline data is comparable with future observations. Additionally, this assessment indicates the need for teaching and skilled observation.

Medication Assessment

The use of both prescription and nonprescription drugs in the home has a major impact on the day to day life of individuals as well as the disease process. It is imperative that a complete medication assessment be done on all clients when admitted to service. The medication regime must also be continuously monitored and evaluated as the patient continues to receive care. The nurse's responsibility is to be aware of this process and report any significant impacts or changes to the physicians, family and patient. All assessment should be done with the view of the patient and family in mind.

Steps

1. Basic Information   All steps in the medication assessment process must be done in light of the patient's current diagnosis and physical assessment. A review of current medications being taken including prescription and nonprescription (OTC) drugs should include:

- Generic and Trade Name
- Dosage
- Method of Administration
- Frequency

- As prescribed
- As taken by the patient
- How long he has taken the drug

- Purpose for the drug
- Interaction—Outcome of the Drug

- Positive outcome—what is "suppose to happen"
- Negative side effects
- Interaction with other drugs the patient is taking

- Name of Physician or Dentist who prescribed drug

2. Drug Allergies   A review of patient's response to certain drugs and ways patient has adjusted. Differentiation must be made from expected side effects and allergic responses. An assessment of food allergies and drug interactions may be necessary.

3. Pharmacy Information   Name, address and phone number of all pharmacies the patient deals with. If possible, the name of specific pharmacist and ability to do home deliveries. Also, it is important to know if the pharmacy has the capacity to check for drug interactions—this may have to be determined directly between the nurse and the pharmacist.

4. Knowledge and Attitude   A review of what the patient knows regarding each medications purpose, dosage, frequency, or side effects. Emphasis should be placed on evaluating the patient's ability to manage medication regimen correctly because of factors such as, eyesight, age, memory difficulties, or confusion about the purpose of the drug. Attitudes regarding fear of side effects, items read in magazines, newspapers, or talking to others with similar diseases or medication should be explored since they have a direct impact on the patient's compliance with the medication regimen.

5. Financial Information   Although this may have been reviewed in previous assessments, you should specifically ask if the patient can pay for or sees the importance of paying for the needed medications. This is especially true if there are many medications or previous information raises the suspicion that the patient may have to choose between medications or other necessities such as food or rent. This is your opportunity to evaluate the patient's need for a referral to other agencies to assist with paying for medications. You may also explore with the patient, physician, and pharmacist if a generic drug can be substituted for a tradename medication.

6. Beliefs   A measurement of the cultural, religious, or social beliefs of the client relative to drugs. Any old medicine, herbal treatments, or advertisement information the client has come in contact with can markedly affect compliance with the regimen. These questions must be asked carefully with the nurse assuming an attitude of helping and understanding not ridicule or judgement.

7. Storage of Medications   A review of how medications are stored in the home. If necessary, an evaluation of the contents of the patient's medicine cabinet can be done with the patient's full cooperation and approval. Often patients have outdated medications and prescription drugs that belong to others.

Nursing Observations and Outcomes

1. Description of the patient's current medication regimen.
2. Indication of patient compliance with the drug regimen.
3. Overview of problems client has with understanding or compliance.
4. Review the patient's ability to learn, that is, can he read, follow written or verbal instructions, and so on.
5. Indication of nurses need to consult with physician or pharmacist regarding possible drug interactions and/or side effects.

Nutrition Assessment

The nutrition status of the individual is a major factor in rehabilitation of the acutely ill patient and in the preservation of function in the chronically ill. Nutrition is clearly not a matter of weight gain and loss, but a factor intimately tied to ambulation, mental acuity, and physical health status. Restoration of tissues, muscle tone, and strength are dependent upon the nourishment supplied to cells through the metabolism of food.

Nutrition assessment in the home must encompass both clinical and practical aspects including keen observations coupled with available laboratory data and information provided by the patient and caregivers. Screening for nutritional problems is clearly a nursing role; but, when the problems and planning become complex, a referral should be made to a registered dietitian. Registered dietitians can be found in hospitals, clinics, community health agencies, and in private practice. Every state has a Dietetic Association with listings of R.D.s and the phone book lists dietitian/nutritionist services identified with an R.D.

Basic information regarding height, changes in weight, and recent or chronic problems that affect eating or digestion need to be gathered in nutritional assessment as well as further assessed during the physical exam. It is also important to determine if vitamin and/or mineral compounds are taken and who shops, cooks, and cleans up. This discussion will usually reveal food preferences, ethnic or cultural cooking, and some clues about social and personal food beliefs.

Steps

1. Baseline Data Establish rapport. Keep in mind that considerable information will be gained that will provide a foundation for teaching if the interview is gently guided rather than just parroting a series of predetermined questions. Listen carefully to the description of *what* is eaten, *when* it is consumed, *how* it is prepared, and *how much* is perceived to be eaten. The patient referred for a therapeutic diet may assume that the diet teaching through the nurse represents taking away part of his lifestyle. Attempts to interject your own ideas and modifications while the patient is talking only reinforces that assumption and reduces the chance of compliance. It is important to be as positive as possible.

2. Food Diary

- Verbal 24-Hour Recall. Having the patient recall what he/she has eaten over the past 24 hours is the most common form of nutritional assessment used since it provides some immediate information for the clinician and a minimal effort by the patient. An estimate of what the patient has eaten is more accurate if the patient shows you the glasses, bowls, or cups used for portions of food.

Remember, it is only an estimate, and should not be the basis of long-term therapy. The 24-hour recall determines if a more precise record is necessary.

- Written Diary. If a more specific description of food patterns and calorie intake is indicated, obtain at least a three-day written diary. This diary must be precise and include:

  - All food, snacks, and beverages consumed.
  - How specific foods were cooked and their amounts.
  - The time of day when the food was eaten.
  - If appropriate, any feelings associated when eating the food.
  - This information can be especially helpful in working with a nutritional consultant.

3. Food Allergies and/or Intolerances   Although not all patients seek out causes for their food intolerances, they are quite clear about recurring discomforts or illness linked with eating certain foods. Consider whether the patients avoidance of offending foods is interfering with the key nutrients. Omission of any of the four food groups in a diet or sources of ascorbic acid, iron, calcium, or other essential nutrients is reason to refer to a dietitian with experience in addressing these problems.

4. Meal Planning   Increasingly, food is being supplied outside the home, in some cases making the kitchen nearly obsolete. The elderly may lean heavily upon TV dinners, take out meals, Meals on Wheels, pizza, and similar foods requiring little or no preparation.

This is an important consideration when assessing patients on special diets. Questions about favorite restaurants, often used TV dinners, or favorite sandwich fillings is important when interventions relative to diet therapy are planned. When the patient is reliant on others for meals, they should be included in the interview so it is clear how and what foods are prepared, and so appropriate choices can be suggested. Encourage eating with others as lone-liness is a powerful appetite suppressant.

5. Concurrent Diet Therapies Past diet therapies are often overlooked during hospitalization and when home care orders are given at discharge. A history of the patient's past diet history should be determined along with the reason for the therapy. New medical conditions or surgical procedures may change past practices, and all involved in the patient's care will need clear instructions on future diet plans at time of admission to home care.

Soon after discharge from a hospital, the diet order is commonly changed or modified on the basis of additional laboratory data. These changes often cause confusion, and the patient may require a personal directive from the physician to accept these orders.

6. Financial Information For the most part, special diets do not cost more than a normal diet. Financial difficulties may arise, however, when the individual on a fixed income experiences large health-care costs. Do not assume the patient's surroundings indicate his ability to pay for food, always address this issue specifically so that assistance can be sought if need be.

7. Community Resources Know the options in the community to assist the patient with meals and financial assistance for food. The patient must be willing to participate, and accurate information should be supplied regarding cost, accessibility, and proximity. Meals On Wheels, elderly hot lunch programs, Food Stamps, community services provided for the hungry, and other support systems in the neighborhood should be explored if necessary.

Nursing Observations and Outcomes The following areas should be clearly documented if the nutritional assessment of the patient was successful:

- Description of patient's current nutritional status with strengths and weaknesses outlined.
- Overview of patient's attitude toward nutrition and diets.

- Assessment of patient's motivation and learning ability.
- Review of previous and potential compliance with regimen.
- Level of needed involvement of family, friends, and community resources.

Assessment Findings Requiring Intervention

Inappropriate Weight Change   Unexplained *weight loss* may result from one or more of the following:

1. Increased metabolic demands from increased mobility.
2. Dilution of food density, especially if soft or liquids comprise the diet.
3. Decreased stomach capacity if TPN or tube feeding has been instituted for a prolonged period.
4. Depression secondary to illness if patient feels he will not recover. Hiding or spitting out food is not uncommon and may go unnoticed.
5. Extreme fatigue which impairs ability to shop/prepare food.
6. Progression of the disease.

Unexplained *weight gain* may result from one or more of the following:

- The patient is not as mobile as he contends.
- Excess calories are consumed, often unknowingly, during recovery.
- Increased appetite secondary to medication effects.
- Increased fluid retention, especially ascites if the patient is poorly nourished. Abdominal girth should be measured when protein and calories are deficient.

Abrupt Changes in Eating Behaviors   Aberrations include:

1. Excessive food consumption
2. Cravings
3. Binging and purging
4. Accumulation of prepared food, resulting in spoilage/vermin hazard

Starvation, self-imposed should be suspected when there is:

1. Lack of food preparation
2. Little or no additions to the garbage over several days
3. Unused cans/packages of nutrition supplements
4. Unwillingness to allow Home Health Aide to prepare food
5. Decreasing weight and unusual amounts of refuse
6. Refusal to be weighed or to remove clothing

Independence In ADLs Assessment— Evaluation for a Home Health Aide

The following index of Independence in ADLs can be helpful in assessing the patient's need for assistance with personal care and the possible placement of a home health aide. Additionally, it can also be used to teach the aide and family future goals and can serve as a guide in documenting the type of care given to the patient. This can mean a clearer picture for reimbursement and quality assurance purposes.

Index of Independence in Activities of Daily Living

The Index of Independence in ADLs is based on an evaluation of the functional independence or dependence of patients in bathing, dressing, going to toilet, transferring, continence, and feeding. Specific definitions of functional independence and dependence appear below the index.

A Independent in feeding, continence, transferring, going to toilet, dressing, and bathing.

B Independent in all but one of these functions.

C Independent in all but bathing and one additional function.

D Independent in all but bathing, dressing, and one additional function.

E Independent in all but bathing, dressing, going to toilet, and one additional function.

F   Independent in all but bathing, dressing, going to toilet, transferring, and one additional function.

G   Dependent in all six functions.

Other   Dependent in at least two functions, but not classifiable as C, D, E, or F.

Independence means without supervision, direction, or active personal assistance, except as specifically noted below. This is based on actual status and not on ability. A patient who refuses to perform a function is considered as not performing the function even though patient is deemed able.

Bathing (Sponge, shower, or tub)

Independent: Assistance only in bathing a single part (as back or disabled extremity) or bathes self completely.

Dependent: Assistance in bathing more than one part of body: assistance in getting in or out of tub or does not bathe self.

Dressing

Independent: Gets clothes from closets and drawers; puts on clothes, outer garments, braces; manages fasteners; act of tying shoes is excluded.

Dependent: Does not dress self or remains partly undressed.

Going to Toilet

Independent: Gets to toilet; gets on and off toilet; arranges clothes; cleans organs of excretion (may manage own bedpan used at night only and may or may not be using mechanical supports).

Dependent: Uses bedpan or commode or receives assistance in getting to and using toilet.

Transfer

Independent: Moves in and out of bed independently and moves in and out of chair independently (may or may not be using mechanical supports).

Dependent: Assistance in moving in or out of bed and/or chair; does not perform one or more transfers.

Continence

Independent: Urination and defecation entirely self-controlled.

Dependent: Partial or total incontinence in urination or defecation; partial or total control by enemas, catheters, or regulated use of urinals and/or bedpans.

Feeding

Independent: Gets food from plate or its equivalent into mouth: (precutting of meat and preparation of food, as buttering bread, are excluded from evaluation).

Dependent: Assistance in act of feeding (*see* above): does not eat at all or parenteral feeding.

SOURCE: Katz, et. al., *JAMA*, Sept. 21, 1963

Evaluation of Functional Activities and Range of Joint Motion— Assessment for Referral to Physical, Speech, or Occupational Therapy

If, upon completing this assessment, the patient is found to be unable to perform the majority of the activities in each category, referral to specific therapy is indicated (*see* page 20).

Bed Activities

1. Ability to change position (move to head of bed, move from side to side, roll from side to side, come to sitting position without assistance).
2. Obtain objects from bedside stand, such as, water glass, tissues, eyeglasses.
3. Ability to give self-care as much as possible, that is, bathing, dental care, and such.

Chair and Wheelchair Activities

1. Ability to get from bed to chair or wheelchair and back.
2. Propel wheelchair.
3. Ability to get from wheelchair to toilet and back.
4. Ability to lock wheelchair.

Standing Activities

1. Bed or chair to standing position and back.
2. Standing balance between two chairs for pivot transfer.
3. Standing balance with assistive device (preparation for crutch walking).

Walking Activities

1. Walk on various levels in home.
2. Walk up and down stairs.
3. Walk up and down curbstones.
4. Walk on uneven surfaces such as stone driveway or yard.

Hygiene Activities

1. Care of teeth, hair, shave, cosmetics, bathing.
2. Manage toilet needs without assistance.
3. Getting into and out of a tub or shower.

Dressing Activities

1. Put on and take off any nightgown, pajama top, shirt, and such.
2. Put on and remove any underclothes.
3. Button and unbutton clothing.
4. Put on and remove hose and shoes.
5. Lace and unlace shoes.
6. Put on and remove braces or other appliances.

Eating Activities

1. Drink from a glass or cup.
2. Cut meat.
3. Eat with fork.
4. Butter bread.

Communication Activities

1. Comprehension—ability to understand verbal/visual clues, follow instructions, and ability to make needs known.
2. Speaking—clear versus slurred speech, appropriate word selection.
3. Eating—Ability to swallow, clean out mouth.

General Activities

1. Turn faucet off and on.
2. Wash and dry dishes.
3. Prepare vegetables.
4. Open bottles.
5. Turn on gas or electric stove.
6. Dusting and polishing.
7. Use of broom, carpet sweeper, or vacuum.
8. Turn door knobs.
9. Switch lights on and off.
10. Pick up objects from floor.
11. Light cigarettes.
12. Take money from small change purse.
13. Any other essential ADLs.

3

Intervention

Planning intervention for the home care patient centers around developing a care plan that identifies how the goals set for the patient will be achieved. This chapter gives guidelines for the preparation of the care plan that can be used when developing plans for all patients in the home.

A care plan has two parts: the basic care plan that addresses common problems observed in every patient regardless of diagnosis, and the individual care plan that identifies specific areas relative to the problems experienced by the patient because of their impairment(s). The first section of this chapter outlines the interventions that are relative to every patient, and the second section addresses the specific problems experienced by the patient based on the type of impairment. Since many patients have several impairments, the home care nurse will need to choose the interventions that fit the individual patient's care plan. All guidelines given in this chapter are phrased in terminology that can be written directly on the patient's care plan.

Section 3-A: The Basic Care Plan

A basic care plan includes interventions that are to be addressed during each home visit regardless of the specific problems the patient is experiencing. The following areas should be a part of *all* care plans devised for home care patients:

- **Monitor Vital Signs**—Include significant indicators of vital signs specific to patient's impairment. (*See* Physical Assessment page 54.)

- **Teach Appropriateness of Physician Interaction**—Instruct patient and family when and how to communicate with the physician.
- **Review Correct Dosage and Administration of Medication Regime**—Observe and teach patient side effects of medications. Since information about medications change rapidly, a current drug reference should also be consulted. (*See* medication interventions for specific impairments.)
- **Instruct in Sound Nutrition and/or Therapeutic Diet**—(*See* nutritional interventions for specific impairments.)

  1. Menus used in the hospital are useful in teaching selections and exchanges.
  2. Modify patient's familiar recipes whenever possible.
  3. Have patient/family review cookbooks at library before purchasing. (Cookbooks references are in the Bibliography.)
  4. Many patients overuse vitamin supplements. Substitute foods high in nutrients whenever possible. (*See* Appendices G and H.)

- **Assess Coping Mechanisms of Patient and Family**—A patient and family's reaction to any illness can follow the five stages of reaction to crisis: denial, bargaining, anger, depression, and acceptance. Speaking to the family alone can often help to uncover problems that can then be dealt with, sometimes through counseling.

- **Assist Patient in Adapting Lifestyle to Disease**
  1. Understand the impact of the illness on current lifestyle.
  2. Find ways to make adaptations as mild as possible—Initiate teaching at a level appropriate to patient's need and understanding.

- **Teach Fundamentals of Aseptic Technique**—All patients cared for in the home and their families need instruction regarding aseptic technique and precautions so the occurrence or spread of infection is prevented. Suggested interventions are:

1. Washing Hands—The most basic and often most overlooked safeguard for patients, family, and home health personnel. Bacteria spread from one patient to another or among the patient and family members are carried most frequently by the hands.
2. Determine the present or potential bacteria and be familiar with the mode and method of transmission before implementing a plan.
3. Teach the family that no matter what disinfectant is used or how long items are soaked, it is mechanical friction that assures items are clean and as germ free as possible.
4. Remember, in the home, the patient/family may use clean technique on some procedures that would require sterile technique in the hospital. In the institutional setting, the patient needs to be protected from the more virulent amount of pathogens, while in the home, the intensity and severity of pathogens is lessened, and the patient has some tolerance to his "own" bacteria. The nurse must always use sterile technique to not introduce pathogens from nurse to patient. (*See* also page 188, Infection Control for the Immunosuppressed Patient.)
5. *See* Procedures Section in Chapter 4 for more information on solutions, disinfectants, and sterilizing equipment in the home.

Section 3-B: Care Plans Specific to Impairments

Care plans specific to various impairments constitute the major portion of this chapter and are a key feature of this handbook. The impairments listed below were chosen because they are the predominant disease conditions seen by home care nurses. These impairments are:

Neurological Functioning
Musculoskeletal Functioning
Cardiac Functioning
Thoracic Functioning
Endocrine Functioning—Diabetes

Circulation
Gastrointestinal-Track Functioning
Urinary-Track Functioning
Skin Integrity
Cancer
Cognitive Functioning

Each section is outlined with terminology that can be written on care plans by using behaviors the nurse can directly perform, teach, supervise, and/or evaluate as care is given. Although not all behaviors are relative to each impairment, the interventions are divided into five areas and outlined as follows:

Introduction to the Impairment—This area describes the impairment giving simple definitions and descriptions which can be shared with patients and families.

Interventions Common to This Impairment—This includes assessments and ongoing evaluations done by the nurse and specific interventions that should be taught to the patient and family.

Additional Interventions Relative to Specific Diseases—Several diseases may be discussed under one impairment section. This area outlines interventions specific to individual diseases.

Medications—The broad interventions relative to medications are described in this area. Detailed medication information was purposely omitted since it is not the scope of this handbook. The home care nurse should frequently use a current drug reference.

Diet–Nutrition—This area outlines clinical and practical nutritional interventions relative to specific diseases. It is useful for nursing assessment and patient teaching.

All interventions listed in this section are guidelines, professional judgement **must** be used in determining which interventions to include based on their relevance to the patient situation. Since many home care patients have more than one diagnosis and/or presenting problem, it is extremely important that suggested interventions in this section be chosen with all factors considered before developing the care plan.

The Patient with Impaired Neurological Functioning

Introduction

There are two types of patients with neurological problems seen in home health care: Those in Group I and those in Group II (a listing follows). The categories are differentiated by the onset of the disease and the patient's rehabilitation potential.

Group I—Cerebral Vascular Accident (CVA), Traumatic Brain Injury (TBI), and Spinal Cord Injury (SCI)

Similarities

Onset:

- Usually sudden followed by a hospital stay, often rehabilitation placement, and then home care.

Rehabilitation Potential:

- Determined by the extent of injury.
- Most gains are made initially and as treatment progresses, slower improvement is seen.
- Lifestyle is significantly different than previous level of functioning—usually results in a new way of living for both patient and family.
- An ongoing therapeutic regime is important for the first few years.

Differences   CVA is approached as a disease of the cardiovascular system with resultant damage to neurological functioning. Interventions focus on rehabilitation of resultant neurological problems associated with CVA are similar to the plan developed for SCI and TBI and will be discussed in this section. Other interventions for the Patient with a CVA can be found in the section entitled, "The Patient with an Impairment of the Cardiac System."

TBI and CVA involve injury to a specific side and/or area of the brain, while SCI has a specific level of spinal lesion identified. The area of the brain involved determines which area of the body is affected, that is, the limbs, trunk, and internal mechanisms such as swallowing, breathing, and elimination. Therefore, an individual treatment/rehabilitation plan must be developed based on the affected area.

Group II—Multiple Sclerosis (MS), Amyotrophic Lateral Sclerosis (ALS), and Parkinson's Disease

Similarities

Onset:

- Gradual—disease process becomes chronic.
- Periods of exacerbation and increased deterioration varying between constant and infrequent remission.

Rehabilitation Potential:

- Focus on preventing further debilitating effects.
- Develop realistic goals so plans can be made and motivation for patient and family can be maintained.
- Lifestyles of both patient and family are significantly changed.

Differences

MS and ALS   Both diseases have increased muscle weakness and decreased coordinated control. Spasticity may or may not be present. As the disease progresses, decreased ability in all activity becomes evident and is compounded by increased difficulty when spasticity is present.

Parkinson's Disease   Has an increased persistence of muscle rigidity with resultant loss of voluntary mobility. As the disease progresses, loss of strength and ROM are the primary debilitating factors. The patient's difficulty is in initiating movement and once moving, keeping coordinated control of the movement, which results in limited independence needed to carry out ADLs.

Interventions for All Neurological Patients

The therapeutic approach to care of the neurological patient is innovative and focused on helping the patient redevelop or modify patterns of movement necessary for normal function. Interventions for these patients are:

— Teach Patient/Family Process of Disease and Rehabilitation Potential

Use information presented under "Similarities" and "Differences."

— Teach Patient/Family Correct Type and Amount of Assistance

- Encourage use of affected areas.
- Promote normal movement by using both sides of the body when appropriate and preventing substitution by other body parts.
- Learn proper positioning before attempting movement—dependent on type of problem.
- Transfer technique, bed mobility, position changes (*see* page 214).
- In caring for patients with Parkinson's, teach the patient to move by rocking. The patient moves by gently rocking back and forth to get up from a sitting or lying position. Once the patient has initiated his own movement, the person assisting can best help by guiding and supporting, eliminating the need to pull, push, or lift the patient.

— Teach Safety Measures

Integrate limitations into current lifestyle and safety techniques into daily activities.

Nutrition—Diet

- Poor mastication can be helped with soft, moistened foods which are chopped, ground, or well cooked.
- Inability to move the bolus of food along the tongue in preparation for swallowing may be eased by use of semi-liquids such as puddings, casseroles, or tender stews.
- Partial throat paralysis needs evaluation to determine what foods are easier to handle. Moist, lubricating foods are needed, but consistencies vary greatly with individuals.
- Evaluate diet relative to Basic Four food groups to determine if types or consistency of foods are decreasing the amount of nutrients the patient is taking.

The Patient with Impaired Musculoskeletal Functioning

Introduction

Interventions for patients with impairments of the musculoskeletal system center around the three areas of immobility, functional barriers, and use of assistive devices.

Interventions for Impaired Musculoskeletal Functioning

Immobility

—Assess for Degenerative Changes in Musculoskeletal Structures Due to Prolonged Bedrest

See Table 3.1.

Table 3.1. Causes of Musculoskeletal Changes in Immobility

Initiating Factors	Initial Changes	Advanced Changes
Poor body alignment	Skeletal malalignment	Skeletal deformities
Restricted use of joints	Limitation of joint mobility Joint stiffness	Ankylosis of joint
Restricted use of muscles	Muscle weakness	Muscle atrophy
	Sustained muscle shortening	Fibrous changes in muscles Muscle contractures

—*Prevent Contractures and Pressure Sores*

- Frequent position changes to prevent contractures and promote circulation.
- Passive and/or active ROM to increase strength.
- Elevation of dependent extremities to prevent edema.
- Transfer techniques using all available assistance from patient.
- Teach family/caregiver proper body mechanics.

—*Teach Safety Regarding Functional Barriers*

- Rearrange furniture if needed to aid patient's movement and safety.
- Remove throw rugs or tape edges to floor to prevent tripping and slipping.
- Remove doors, install ramps, and/or rails, if necessary.
- Rearrange closets, cabinets, and drawers.

—*Teach Use of Assistive Devices* (See also page 225)

Walker Used when decrease in balance, no weight bearing on one extremity or disability or weakness of one or both lower extremities.

Walker Safety:
- Always place all four legs of the walker on the floor at the same time.
- Progress walker so the back legs of the walker are just ahead of patient's toes.
- Step only halfway into the walker to prevent loss of balance backwards.
- Encourage leaning forward on the walker for increased stability.

Crutches   Same as above, only patient has good balance.

Crutch Safety:
- Have good balance upon standing before beginning appropriate gait pattern.
- If using two crutches, remember to leave space wide enough to fit body through.

Cane   Used with patients with fair balance, weakness in one lower extremity or partial weight bearing of one lower extremity.

Cane Safety:
- Progress forward and to the side greater than six inches to prevent tripping over the cane, especially if using a quad cane.
- Longer legs of quad cane are always pointed away from the body if on level flooring or heading down the stairs for maximum stability.

Wheelchair   Used in the following situations:

1. Patients with tendency toward edema—should have elevating leg rests.
2. Patients with difficulty transferring — removable leg rests and arm rests to allow close proximity between wheelchair and other surfaces.
3. If wheelchair is too wide to pass through doorways or halls, a device called "Sx-Reduce-A-Width" can reduce the width of a wheelchair as much as four inches to get through a doorway and the W/C then returns to normal size. Check with a DME supplier for more information.

Hospital Bed   Used to encourage normal position changes, ease caregiver's work, and to assist with mobility. A trapeze should be used only when patient needs assistance moving in bed.

Sling   Used for painful or subluxated shoulder and for flaccid upper extremity to increased control of total body movements.

Lift Bars, Commode, Tub Rails, and Tub Seat   These should be used after careful evaluation by a physical or occupational therapist who can judge the specific type of equipment needed and its placement. Erroneous judgment in this area can lead to unneeded expense, ineffective use by the patient, and damage to walls of a home.

—Teach Transfer Techniques

Assess bed, seat, and wheelchair height for optimum transfers (see page 217 for specific transfer techniques).

Nutrition—Diet

For Immobile Patients

- Prevent excessive weight gain by controlling calories and assisting patient to find other areas of enjoyment so food does not become a focal point.
- The immobile patient will have more difficulty in weight control, and success needs to be measured by how well the patient has maintained his current weight or slowed down weight gain rather than expecting a weight loss.
- Teach family importance of weight control and its effect on transferring and lifting of patient. Entire family may need to reduce intake of calories and not eat in front of patient to assist in controlling weight.
- Constipation is a major problem—a high-fiber diet, increase in fluids, and eating cooked fruits and vegetables will help in the formation of softer stools.

For Immobile Patients with Broken Bones

- A high-protein, high-nutrient diet is needed for healing; therefore, calories must be cut from desserts, fats, and "empty calories."
- Calcium in the diet should be increased with dairy or supplemental products. Milk intolerant patients should use nondairy nutritional supplements fortified with calcium until the break is well healed. (See Appendix J.)
- Use of a calcium supplement should continue to be used to ensure that the elements for normal bone matrix are provided.

The Patient with Impaired Cardiac Functioning

Introduction

As the leading cause of death in the United States, heart disease represents a significant portion of the home care caseload. The main cardiac diseases requiring follow-up in the home and the divisions of this section are:

1. Cerebral vascular accident (CVA).
2. Coronary artery disease, including angina and congestive heart failure (CHF).
3. Hypertension.

As with other disease conditions, the physiology of the disease indicates the patient's symptoms. The most common are:

Right-Sided Heart Failure: Systemic symptoms due to inefficiency of the right ventricle and systemic vascular congestion.

Left-Sided Heart Disease: Pulmonary problems due to inefficient left ventricular function and pulmonary congestion.

Interventions for All Cardiac Patients

—*Cardiac Assessment Including Vital Signs*

- A thorough cardiothoracic assessment is indicated for all cardiac patients on every visit. Refer to Physical Assessment, page 74, for a thorough discussion on the procedure.
- Teach patient/family how to take a pulse.

  1. Establish a baseline pulse for comparison.
  2. Show how to "feel" and count radial pulse.
  3. Take a resting pulse, that is, just before getting out of bed each morning.
  4. Count pulse for one full minute.
  5. Avoid taking carotid pulse as it may cause arrhythmias or asystole.
  6. Keep a record of pulse rates and report changes in rate or quality.

—*Assess for Fluctuations in Weight*

- Develop way to differentiate increase weight from edema and excess caloric intake.
- Weigh on a consistent scale.
- Frequency of weight assessment is determined by the severity of cardiac involvement. The usual guidelines are:

  - Weigh Daily—Those patients whose small weight gain from edema results in acute CHF, and/or those patients on intense diuretic therapy.
  - Weigh Weekly or Biweekly—Those patients less labile. If overweight, a reducing diet inclusive of other dietary restrictions is indicated. If weight is

ideal, efforts must be taken to maintain weight and guard against weight gain in the face of reduced exercise.

—Monitor for Edema

- Edema is found most commonly in lower extremities.
- Any part of the body that is dependent should be assessed for edema. For example, the patient on bedrest can have sacral edema rather than in the legs.
- Use accurate and consistent measures of edema by following procedures outlined in the "Physical Assessment" section of Chapter 2. The use of 1+ to 4+ is ambiguous, and it is impossible to be consistent among health providers.

—Monitor Amount and Type of Exercise

- Although various amounts of fatigue are present in all cardiac patients, it is important to stress an exercise plan.
- If the patient is in a formal cardiac rehabilitation program, reinforce exercise components within guidelines, refer to Physical Therapist as necessary.
- Be sure patient understands accurate assessment of amount of activity performed. Environmental factors such as steps, ramps, and reaching may result in more exertion than allowed while the patient does not perceive that as exercise.

—Assess Patient/Family Emotional Status

- Since the heart is seen as the center of life and feeling, severe emotional stress is associated with the diagnosis, role loss, and treatment modality.
- Family response to the illness can increase patient's stress and feelings of worthlessness.

- Observation of the family interactions as well as speaking to the patient and family members separately can help to support that they are not alone in their feelings and may need a mutual support group.

—Teach Reduction of Complicating Factors

- Cessation of smoking.
- Decrease in alcohol intake.
- A more relaxed lifestyle, using relaxation techniques, if necessary. (See Relaxation Techniques, page 210.)

—Monitor and Teach Importance of Bowel Regime

Establish normal bowel regime to prevent constipation and straining of bowel movements. (See Establishing a Bowel Regimen, page 156.)

—Monitor Intake and Output

- A gross assessment of intake and output is sufficient in most patients.
- If a more rigorous assessment is indicated, specific measurements should be recorded daily. The initiation of intake and output can be ordered by the physician or the home care nurse. (See Table of Equivalents in Appendix O.)

Interventions for Specific Cardiac Diseases

Cerebral Vascular Accident (CVA)

The following will focus on the medical management of the underlying disease causing a CVA. Rehabilitation relative to the neurological damage suffered by a CVA can

be found in the section "The Patient with Impaired Neurological Functioning."

—*Monitor for Signs, Symptoms, and Complications of Recurrence of the Disease*

Headache—Monitor frequency, severity and pattern of
the headache. Often, an intermittent headache is a
bothersome sequelae of a stroke and often the fore-
runner of an impending new one. Isolated headaches
are not a major concern.

Motor Deficits—Ongoing evaluation of changes in motor deficits relative to ongoing need for appropriate
physical, speech, or occupational therapy.

Coronary Artery Disease—Congestive Heart Failure—Angina

—*Monitor Chest Pain*

- Measure the amount of exertion it takes to initiate the
  pain.
- How often is it happening?
- Measure the type—that is, crushing, burning, dull,
  sharp, choking, and so on.
- How long does an episode last?
- Identify the precipitating factors.
- Assess relieving factors for the episode.
- Document the amount and type of medication used
  to relieve the episode.

—*Assess Respiratory Status*

Thoroughly assess respiratory status and involvement
on each visit. Refer to Physical Assessment Section, page
68, for discussion of this procedure.

Hypertension

—*Monitor for Signs, Symptoms, and Complications of the Disease*

- **Headache**—Many patients may not experience a headache and be having a hypertensive crisis. If headaches do occur, determine the frequency, severity, and pattern and determine with patient and physician if linked to rises in blood pressure.
- **Nosebleeds**—Many patients experience nosebleeds when their B/P is elevated. Instruct in how to care for a nosebleed and how to monitor for hypertension.
- Teach patient or family procedure for taking blood pressure. Kits are available commercially and are the accurate way to monitor B/P at various times during day.

Medications

The quantity, use, and dose of cardiac medications changes frequently and varies in different parts of the country. For this reason, the nurse is asked to consult a drug reference, the patient's physician, and pharmacist when questions arise on specific medication interventions for the cardiac patient. The following tips should be used when discussing cardiac medications with a patient to assure prescribed medications are taken appropriately:

- Hypertensive patients may tend to stop taking medications if unpleasant side effects occur. Since hypertension is asymptomatic, the patient needs to be assured that the medication is being effective in lowering his B/P even though he doesn't "feel" any better.
- Of course, any unusual or significant side effects should be reported to the physician immediately.
- Often cardiac patients have numerous pills that look alike, especially ones that are small and white. Always ask the patient how they are *supposed* to take the medication and how they *actually* take it and clarify

if there is any confusion about which pill is which.
There are commercial products available to assist patients in taking medication at the proper times. (*See*
page 242 for helpful hints regarding medications.)
- Generic medications can often be substituted for brand-
name drugs and patients may become more compliant
if medication costs less. Check with physician and
pharmacist if substitutions can be made.

Nutrition—Diet

—Teach Sodium-Restricted Diet as Ordered

- Stress the positive aspects of the diet, emphasizing
the allowed foods rather than the foods not to use.
- Be familiar with new products which incorporate lower
sodium content and reduced cholesterol/saturated fat
content. Lists of allowable foods and ones to avoid
can be found in Appendix E.
- Salt substitutes should only be used if ordered by the
physician since medication and electrolyte interactions can occur with salt substitutes.
- Encourage the use of various spices other than salt in
cooking.
- Teach the patient with a mild sodium restriction (2-
4 gm/day) guidelines for reading labels:

  —Bread and cereal products should contain 200 mg
  or less of sodium per serving to be acceptable.
  —Lightly salted canned vegetables should be kept to
  150 mg/serving.
  —Lightly salted margarine helps to keep sodium intake low.
  —Lightly salted prepared food should not exceed more
  than one serving/day. Use these guidelines:

    *Lightly salted turkey breast (not turkey roll)
    *Fresh roast beef from the deli, not ones in cryovac
    packages.
    *TV dinners are available with less than 750 mg of
    sodium and can be used if patient is willing to

carefully avoid other extra sodium sources that day.

*Other convenience food with high-sodium content can be used *only* with permission from the physician and should be accompanied by other food with minimal levels of sodium to prevent undue fluid accumulation.

—Teach Ongoing Expectations for Diet and Medications

- Secondary effects of medications should be addressed early in treatment. Many patients with complex medication schedules experience alterations in taste, intolerance of cooking aromas, gastrointestinal discomfort, early satiety, and poor appetite. Small, frequent meals with warm or cool food may alleviate some of this distress.
- As the disease progresses, multiple nutrition problems can arise:

  1. Increasing restrictions of sodium and fluids may lead to weight loss and tissue wasting if the patient is eating poorly.
  2. Well-seasoned, but unsalted food can be used for the family too, relieving the burden of the caregiver.
  3. Small meals with snacks or liquid nutritional supplements between meals will boost calorie and protein intake.

The Patient with Impaired Thoracic Functioning

Introduction

Some thoracic diseases are related to cardiac function- ing and have been outlined in the section on "Impaired Cardiac Functioning." Thoracic disease discussed in this section will focus on obstructive disease—COPD and asthma—and infectious diseases—bronchitis and pneu- monia. Even though these diseases are varied in etiology and pathology, the interventions are similar.

Interventions for All Respiratory Patients

—*Monitor and Teach Patient Signs and Symptoms of Infection*

- Respiratory rate and temperature are early indicators of infection.
- Sputum should be monitored for amount, color, and character. Green sputum is an indication of infection and should be reported to the physician.
- Coughing should be encouraged if it is productive and helps clear phlegm from the lungs. If the cough is bothersome and nonproductive, the physician should determine the intervention. Thoracic patients should only use cough suppressants prescribed by the phy- sician.
- Fluids should be encouraged to thin secretions, unless contraindicated.
- On every visit, a thorough lung assessment is indi- cated (*see* page 68).

—*Monitor and Teach Methods Relative to Activity*

- Assess activity tolerance.
- Assess and teach need for organizing activities and arranging home environment for maximum efficiency. A referral for physical or occupational therapy is often helpful.
- Determine need for assistance in the home for personal care and ADLs. Encourage independence as tolerated. (*See* ADL assessment guidelines, page 107.)
- Determine need for assistive devices.
- Teach energy conservation, breathing, and relaxation techniques as ordered and appropriate (*see* page 209).

—*Teach Reduction of Risk Factors*

- Refer to American Lung Association for assistance in smoking cessation or other needs of patient—contact local chapter for information. Contact physician for nicotene gum to focus on decrease of smoking if abstinence is not possible.
- Limit exposure to URIs from family and friends and contact with cold weather.
- Have paper bag or lined trash basket close to patient for disposal of tissues that contain phlegm.
- Cover mouth when coughing and sneezing.
- Avoid extreme weather conditions which cause allergic reactions.
- Severe cold and heat will usually cause exacerbation of respiratory symptoms
- Housepets with long hair and/or fur or items that tend to collect dust should be kept away from patient's living area and belongings.

—*Teach Use of Oxygen in the Home (If Ordered)*

- The need for oxygen as compared to the use and physician's order should be monitored closely with the patient.

- Instruct patient on the problems incurred when too much oxygen is used as compared to what is needed.
- Use water-soluble lubricant under nose when using nasal cannula.
- Safety precautions to prevent explosion and fire in areas where oxygen is used are:

  —No smoking, lighted matches, or cigarette lighters.
  —The room should be kept free of static electricity to avoid sparks. This can be accomplished by:

  1. Using a vaporizer to raise the humidity level.
  2. Management of bed linens—no electric blankets, polyester or nylon bedspreads, blankets, sheets, or pillowcases. Use only cotton, muslin or nonstatic materials.
  3. Clothing management—no nylon gowns or pajamas, use only nonstatic materials while oxygen is in use.

—Teach Use of Ventilation Devices (If Ordered)

- Be sure patient/family are familiar with operation of all devices used including schedule of periodic cleaning.
- An emergency plan should be developed, and everyone in the family should be aware of it. Relevant phone numbers should be handy.
- Some devices require the administration of medication into the machine. Careful instruction regarding dose and cleanliness should be monitored.

—Monitor Intake and Output

- Adequate fluid intake is essential for hydration and to reduce the viscosity of respiratory secretions provided there are no contraindications present from a secondary diagnosis.
- A fluid intake of at least one quart (948 mL) per day

is desirable. All fluids are suitable except those which have a milk base as they tend to increase viscosity of phlegm.

- If diuretics or fluid restrictions are ordered, teach "hints" on how to limit fluids and still meet needs. (*See* page 246.)

Medications

See Table 3.2.

Table 3.2. Commonly Used Nebulized Drugs

Drug	Indications	Nursing Implications
	Bronchodilators & Decongestants	
Racemic epinephrine	Bronchospasm in asthma or bronchitis, laryngeal, or tracheal edema	Extreme cautions with elderly or patients having thyroid or heart disease. Can cause N&V, elevated B/P, headache.
Isoproterenol	Bronchospasm	Same as above. Can cause arrhythmias, tremors, excitement, and tachycardia.
Isotharine	Bronchospasm	Although safer than preceeding drugs, use caution in patients with heart disease.
Terbutaline	Bronchospasm	Rare

(Continued)

Table 3.2—Continued

Proteolytics

Acetylcysteine	Abnormally thick or inspissated secretions in airways.	Use with caution with asthma or other bronchospastic disorders. Use with bronchodilator. Use with caution in patients who can't cough up secretions.

Antifoaming Agents

Ethyl alcohol	Pulmonary edema due to left ventricular failure	None

Cortiosteroids

Beclomethasone	Patients with steroid-dependent asthma.	Not used in patients with sattus asthmaticus or other acute episode of asthma.

Miscellaneous

Cromolyn sodium		Not used in patients with status asthmaticus or other acute episode of asthma; may have to be given in combination with bronchodilator if brings on bronchospasm.

SOURCE: Adapted from *The Lippincott Manual of Nursing Practice, 3rd Edition.* Used with Permission. J. B. Lippincott, Philadelphia, Penn., 1982.

Diet—Nutrition

- Calorie control may be needed for the individual who is unable to exercise vigorously.
- The patient with far advanced disease may become anorectic, since fatigue is a potent appetite depressant. Small, frequent meals requiring little chewing can preserve precious energy.

The Patient with Impaired Functioning of the Endocrine System: Diabetes

Introduction

Few disease conditions rival diabetes for its impact on every body system and the self-concept of the patient. Because of the colliding forces prevalent in such patients, caring for the diabetic in the home becomes a significant challenge.

Three types of diabetic patients are seen by home health agencies: the newly diagnosed, the new insulin-dependent patient with an acute exacerbation, and the chronic diabetic. A newly diagnosed diabetic or a patient new to insulin requires an inclusive teaching plan addressing both the physiological and psychological aspects of the diagnosis. Likewise, it is important to remember that even a long standing diabetic, one who has had the disease for several years, may need the same level of intervention and reinforcement. Often, instructions are forgotten or lose their impact over the years, and the patient may be more receptive to learning at the latter stage of his illness when the effects of the disease are more apparent.

Interventions Specific to All Diabetics

—Assess and Teach Monitoring of Skin Condition—Foot Care

See Procedures for Foot Care, page 203.

—Monitor and Teach Blood and Urine Testing

Blood Testing

- Instruct patient on importance of having blood tests performed as ordered.
- If home blood-glucose monitoring device is used, review procedure and intrepretation based on the specific unit used.
- Evaluate results of blood tests performed at laboratory (see Appendix C.)
- Teach patient to keep a written record of blood and urine results for review on subsequent visits and for reporting to the physician.

Urine Testing

- Test urine as much as four times per day depending on orders and patient need.
- Evaluate patient's technique and result of urine testing. Things to remember when doing a urine test:

  1. Always use a fresh urine sample, do not use the first voided specimen in the morning as invalid results may occur.
  2. If tablets are used for testing, never touch them with wet fingers. This activates the chemicals and could burn the skin.
  3. The procedure and waiting time for each test is:

     Clinitest: 5 drops of urine, 10 drops of water, tablet; read in 15 seconds.
     Clinitest: 2 drops of urine, 10 drops of water, tablet; read in 15 seconds.

Clinistix: Dip the stix and hold strip horizontal; read in 10 seconds.

Acetest: Place 1 drop of urine directly on tablet; wait 30 seconds.

Ketostix: Dip the stix in urine and hold strip horizontal; read in 15 seconds.

Tes-Tape: Use about 1.5 inch; dip one end in urine for 2 seconds, wait 60 seconds and read.

See Table 3.3 for a comparison of urine tests.

Table 3.3. Comparison of Urine Tests

Method	0%	0.5%	1%	2%	3%	4%	5%
Clinitest							
two-drop	N	1+	2+	3+	4+		5+
five-drop	N T	1+	2+	3+	4+		
Diastix	N T	1+	2+	3+			
Benedict's	N	1+		2+	3+	4+	
Tes-Tape		1+	2+	3+	4+		
Clinistix	N	Light means ¼% or less;					
		Dark means ½% or more;					
		Medium means between ¼% & ½%					

NOTE: Percent (%) = gm/100 mL; N = normal; T = trace.
Hoole, Axalla J., R. Greenberg, C. Glenn Pickard, *Patient Care Guidelines for Nurse Practitioners, 2nd Edition.* Copyright © 1982 by Axalla J. Hoole, Robert A. Greenberg, and C. Glen Pickard, Jr; Boston: Little, Brown and Company, 1982. Used with Permission.

—*Teach Patient/Family Sick-Day Routine*

Instruct patient to do the following when they are ill:

- Continue to take insulin or oral agents during the illness.
- Monitoring urine and blood testing is especially important during this time.
- Force fluids and eat if at all possible. If unable to eat solid food, liquids high in glucose should be given. Usually orange juice with 2 teaspoons sugar is given but any juice with added sugar may be used.

—Instruct on the Importance of Identification Card

All diabetics should wear an identification bracelet and carry a medic alert card, which can be obtained through the local chapter of the American Diabetic Association and at pharmacies.

—Teach Signs, Symptoms, and Treatment of Hypo- and Hyperglycemia

Hypoglycemia (Insulin Shock)

Symptoms

- Rapid onset as result of sudden decrease in blood sugar (usually below 50 mg/dL).
- Sweating, tremor, pallor, tachycardia, palpitation, nervousness—from release of adrenalin from CNS.
- Headache, lightheadedness, confusion, emotional changes, memory lapses, numbness of lips and tongue, slurred speech, lack of coordination, staggering gait, double vision, drowsiness, convulsions, coma—from depression of the CNS when blood glucose falls rapidly.

Treatment

- Give some form of sugar orally such as orange juice, candy, or lump of sugar.
- Teach patients to carry carbohydrate with them at all times.
- Instruct family that nothing should be given by mouth if patient is unconscious; patient should be taken to an emergency room.
- Maintain regular schedule of diet, exercise, and insulin.
- Extra food should be taken before unusual physical exertion.

Hyperglycemia (Ketoacidosis & Diabetic Coma)

Signs and Symptoms

- Onset is gradual.
- Ketones and sugar will appear in the urine.
- Early manifestations: polyuria, polydipsia, fatigue, malaise, drowsiness, anorexia, headache, abdominal pains, muscle cramps, nausea, vomiting, constipation.
- Later manifestations: Kussmaul breathing (very deep respiratory movements).
- Sweet, fruity breath, hypotension, weak, thready pulse, and in later stages, stupor and coma.

Treatment

- Contact primary care provider and, if unable to do so in a reasonable time, go to the hospital.
- Drink only fluids without sugar such as tea, broth, and diet soda.

Medication

Oral Hypoglycemic Agents

Many patients have impaired insulin production levels and can be treated effectively with proper diet, exercise, and oral agents rather than injections of insulin. These patients require the same interventions relative to foot care, urine testing, and other areas of concern for the diabetic. Interventions relative to oral agents center around monitoring side effects and effect of the medication on symptoms of the disease.

—*Teach/Instruct Specifics About Insulin*

Action

Preparations used to replace insulin production in humans are commonly extracted from beef or pork pancreas;

beef is the least allergic and is, therefore, more commonly used. In addition to regular insulin, various modified forms of insulin are available as well as new types of insulin developed that are even less allergenic. Insulins are classified as:

1. Rapid acting
2. Intermediate acting
3. Long acting

Individual response to insulin varies and is affected by diet, exercise, concomitant drug therapy, and other factors. Table 3.4 indicates the onset, peak, and duration of insulin given by subcutaneous injection.

Table 3.4. Onset, Peak, and Duration of Action of Insulin

Insulin	Onset (hr)	Peak (hr)	Duration (hr)
Rapid acting			
Insulin injection (regular)	0.5–1	2–5	6–8
Prompt insulin zinc suspension (such as, Semilente)	0.5–1.5	5–10	6–8
Intermediate acting			
Isophane insulin suspension (such as, NPH)	1–1.5	8–12	24
Insulin zinc suspension (such as, Lente)	1–2.5	7–15	24
Long acting			
Protamine zinc insulin suspension (such as, PZI)	4–8	14–20	36
Extended insulin zinc suspension (such as, Ultralente)	4–8	10–30	>36

Administration and Dosage

- The number, size of dose, and time of administration are determined by close medical supervision.

- Regular insulin is given 15–30 minutes before a meal; longer-acting preparations are usually given before breakfast.
- Rotate sites of administration to prevent lipodystrophy.
- Vials of insulin suspensions should be rotated several times before withdrawing each dose to ensure uniform suspension. Avoid vigorous shaking.
- Always use the syringe that matches the strength of insulin and use the same type and brand of syringe to avoid dosage errors.
- Do not change the dosage, strength, brand, or mixture of insulin without consulting the physician.

Storage

- Insulin preparations are stable at room temperature. Insulin should be stored in a cool place, preferably the refrigerator.
- Current research indicates insulin prefilled in plastic or glass syringes is considered stable for 1 week under refrigeration. Eli Lilly advocates this conservative recommendation based on the factor of sterility rather than stability. Since there is no way to determine the care used in prefilling syringes, it is felt this is the preferable policy.

Mixing Various Types of Insulin

- Neutral regular insulin may be mixed with crystalline PZI insulin in any proportion. Semilente, Ultralente, and Lente insulins may also be combined.
- If regular insulin is mixed with NPH or with Lente, the effect of giving the two separately is only achieved if given within 5 minutes of mixing; after this time the mixture is unstable.
- Draw the shorter-acting insulin first. This is important to avoid contaminating the vial and, thus, slowing the action time of future doses. Contaminating one insulin with another can alter the action of the contaminated insulin.

Nutrition—Diet

- Teach use of diabetic exchange diets, if ordered, including ways of adjusting cultural and personal recipes to exchange lists. A chart of the exchanges found on diabetic diets is included in Appendix F.
- Refer to sources of information on food products; local market availability of diet items and cookbooks (See Bibliography) can help patient/family see that a wider range of foods can be used than was believed. These aides also assist in better compliance with diet restrictions and integration into the family meals.
- Teach that special diet food need not be purchased. Often new or unstable chronic diabetics purchase the expensive prepared food labeled "dietitic." A great deal of money can be saved by purchasing food packed in its own juice or water and rinsing the food under water before cooking or eating.
- Diet diaries are helpful in assessing whether compliance is the problem responsible for elevated blood sugar levels. Three to five days of precise records of all foods and beverages as well as the types of food, amount, method of preparation, and spacing of meals must be included.
- Use of a 24-hour recall coupled with an estimate of foods purchased and consumed weekly will also give indication of food practices.

The Patient with Impaired Circulation

Introduction

The most frequent disease related to impaired circulation requiring home health care is peripheral vascular disease which covers the various diseases of phlebitis, thrombophlebitis, phlebothrombosis, arteriosclerosis, and athrosclerosis. These conditions can often result in stasis ulcers and/or amputations. Additionally, the neuropathy experienced by diabetics can also result in amputations. This section will cover the interventions specific to these patients and will focus on the patient with PVD and amputations.

Interventions Specific to Peripheral Vascular Disease

—*Monitor/Teach Prevention of Further Impairment*

- Instruct on keeping involved extremities warm and protected from injury.
- Since extremities with impaired circulation cannot sense the extent of heat and cold, bath water should be checked carefully with the hand to prevent heat injury.
- Deliberate skin and foot care (*see* page 203).
- Heating pads and hot water bottles should not be used.
- Advise against wearing restrictive garments such as garters, belts, tight pantyhose, and panty girdles.
- Teach the dangers of smoking and how these dangers affect the constriction of blood vessels.
- Walking is the best form of exercise; otherwise, active or passive exercise is recommended.

—*Observe/Teach Signs and Symptoms of Circulatory Disturbances*

- Pain in the extremity—note whether at rest, with limited activity, or with more pronounced exercise.
- Color changes of the skin or nails—pallor, pinkness rubor, and cyanosis.
- Impaired or peculiar growth of nails.
- Shiny, taut skin.
- Discrepancy in size of one extremity as compared to the opposite one.
- Enlarged veins or abnormal pulsations of veins.
- Temperature variation—abnormally cold or abnormally warm.
- Ulcerations, necrosis, or gangrene.

—*Provide and Teach Care of Stasis Ulcers*

Care is directed as ordered by physician and follows procedure for all wound care as outlined in the section, The Patient with Impaired Skin Integrity, page 171.

Medications

—*Teach Patient Guidelines for Anticoagulant Therapy*

- Take medication same time every day and exactly in the dosage prescribed.
- Wear a bracelet or carry a card indicating that anticoagulants are being taken and name and phone number of physician.
- Avoid taking any other medications without first checking with physician. Particularly check about taking vitamins, aspirin, mineral oil, cold medicines, antibiotics, and phenylbutazone (Butazolidin).
- Recognize importance of frequent blood testing.

—Teach Warning Signs that Should Be Reported Immediately

- Excessive bleeding that does not stop quickly (a small cut, brushing teeth, a nosebleed).
- Skin discoloration or bruises that appear suddenly.
- Black or bloody bowel movements—check with Hemoccult if necessary.
- Blood in urine.
- Faintness, dizziness, or unusual weakness.

Interventions Specific to Amputations

Lower extremity amputation occurs more frequently than upper extremity. The following interventions can be used for all amputated patients:

—Teach Positioning to Prevent Hip and/or Knee Contractures

- Lie prone one to two times per day and increase time tolerance to 30 minutes.
- Avoid using a pillow under knee—elevate below the knee.
- Provide support under abdomen. (See "Bed Positioning" page 214.)

—Teach Stump Wrapping Procedure

Remember: This is not a dressing, but a pressure wrap designed to mold the stump in the proper shape so a prosthesis may be fitted successfully.

Below Knee Amputation

- All patients are candidates for prosthetic usage unless specifically stated and must wear a shrinker and/or ace bandage (4-6 in.) at all times.

- The wrap should be removed every 4-6 hr (including nighttime), skin should be checked, and the wrap should be reapplied.
- If an oozing wound is present on the stump, apply one 4x4 in. gauze bandage only; if dry scab is present, no gauze is needed. Never put roller gauze under a shrinker/ace bandage.
- Wrap on a diagonal as illustrated in Figure 3.1.
- Apply significant pressure distally and decrease as you go proximally, continuing to above the knee. This method allows for proper venous return.

Above Knee Amputation

Primary weight-bearing area for an above knee amputation is the ischial tuberosity; therefore, stump wrapping is somewhat different than for a below knee amputation. Problems arise when the patient is ace wrapped or uses a shrinker and the medial aspect of the wrap folds down, thus leaving a medial fleshy roll protruding. This fleshy roll can result in an improper socket fit and a prosthesis that cannot be used. It is *essential* that the stump be wrapped as follows:

- The Ace wrap (6 in. wide) is secured by a hip spica as illustrated in Figure 3.2.
- Wrap on the diagonal and apply significant pressure distally and decrease as you go proximally.
- An index card with moleskin on it can be placed over the medial thigh to prevent rolling of the bandage.
- If the patient uses an AK shrinker, be sure the belt is fastened securely and passes through all the belt loops.

—*Encourage Movement*

See ROM exercises, page 218.

—*Teach Gait Training*

See Gait Training, page 226.

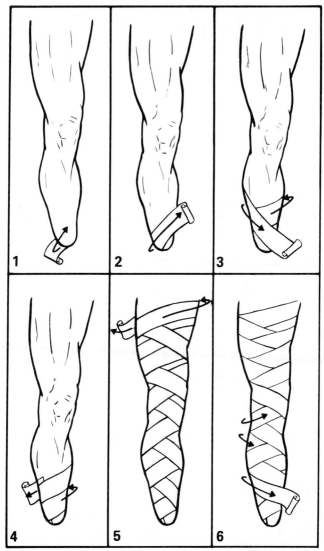

Figure 3.1. Stump wrapping procedure for below knee amputation.

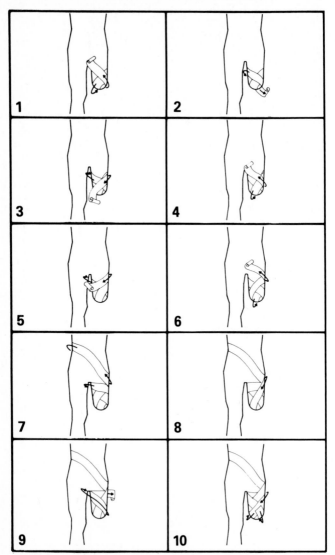

Figure 3.2. Stump wrapping procedure for above knee amputation.

The Patient with Impaired Gastrointestinal Functioning

Introduction

Impairments of the GI tract can be the patient's primary diagnosis or secondary to their main condition, treatment, or medication side effect. Since the GI System has numerous sections, each will be dealt with separately; commonalities for all patients with GI disturbances will also be covered. The GI tract is a continuous system; each part must be evaluated as interventions are planned and evaluated.

The Mouth

The most common mouth problems are:

- Poor dentition—results from poor oral health, history of oral problems with resultant caries, gum disease, missing teeth, and ill-fitting dentures. Such problems can result in loss of nutrients since these patients often choose bland and refined foods low in nutrients such as tea and toast rather than grinding foods that are more nutritional.
- Dryness—side effects of medications, use of oxygen, mouth breathing, lack of humidity in room, and previous radiation to head and neck.
- Neuromuscular problems—affect ability to chew/swallow and can affect the function of the esophagus; this can also affect ability of patient to wear dentures.
- Physical blockage—Polyps or structures can occur at the same time as previous problems or alone.

Interventions Specific to the Mouth

—Teach Patient/Family Importance of Good Dental Care

- Refer for dental care. Resources in many communities provide dental care at reduced or low cost.
- Encourage to start and follow through with dental care.
- Teach the importance of wearing dentures and ways to make fit more comfortable and secure.

—Teach Patient/Family Principles of Good Oral Hygiene

- If dryness is a problem, establish cause.
- If dryness is a side effect of medication, instruct on use of artificial saliva lubricant, many of which are on the market.
- If dehyrdation is the problem, increase oral fluids.
- If patient is a mouth breather or user of oxygen, provide humidity in room.
- If poor oral care is due to health practices, disease condition, or any of the reasons just listed, the following suggestions for cleaning and mouthwashes can be taught:

  —Frequency of cleaning the oral cavity is dependent on the needs of the patient, but once a day is minimum.
  —Cleaning is best done by friction either by toothbrush or by massaging the gums and teeth with gentle pressure of the finger and/or a cotton swab or moist gauze.
  —Rinsing must be done after cleaning to irrigate the tissues. If rinsing can't be done by the patient, the caregiver should be taught irrigation with a large hypodermic syringe or bulb syringe if patient can manage fluids without choking. Irrigate cautiously in the patient with a compromised airway.
  —A lubricant should be applied to exposed extraoral tissue only.

—Mouthwashes can either be purchased commercially or prepared in the home. Some useful preparations for mouthwash are:

Sodium chloride solution (0.9%)—1 teaspoon salt to 1 pint tepid water. Monitor sodium intake in hypertensive patients.

Sodium bicarbonate—1 teaspoon sodium bicarbonate to 1 pint tepid water. Monitor sodium intake in hypertensive patients.

Hydrogen peroxide—Equal parts hydrogen peroxide (U.S.P. 3%) and water, saline (0.9%) or mouthwash mixed just prior to use and used minimum of 1.5 min. If used frequently, contact physician or dentist. Should not be used with patients who have fresh granulation surfaces in the mouth.

Glycerin—Should be mixed with lemon juice in a 1:1 proportion, then used as a softener rather than a cleaner, and rinsed with clear water after using. When used over a long period of time, lemon juice can be harmful to the enamel of the teeth, and glycerin can dry mouth tissue and be painful to broken mucosa. This preparation, although widely used, is not suitable for intraoral use.

Petroleum—Used on the lips and external skin of mouth to prevent drying. Helpful in patient who is dehydrated or mouthbreathing.

The Esophagus and Stomach

The most common problems affecting the stomach and esophagus are:

- Side effects of medications or treatments.
- High level of stress, which results in swallowing air, eating too rapidly, and going for long periods of time without food.
- Poor eating habits—slouching while eating, eating on the run, and eating too many fats and not enough roughage and nutritional foods.
- Underlying physiological problems such as esophageal reflux or hiatal hernia.

Interventions Specific to the Esophagus and Stomach

Nutrition—Diet

—Teach Proper Eating Habits

* Eat at prescribed times and sit down in a relaxed atmosphere.
* Eat slowly, chew food well, and sit up properly so food will flow down the esophagus smoothly.
* Decrease amount of fats in diet. Carbohydrates are digested first, proteins second, and fats take the longest time to exit the stomach.
* Determine what foods cause the most problems. Spicy food is often irritating. Fruits and other high acid food should not be eaten by themselves between meals unless antacids or buffering products are included. Prior to sleep, food should be avoided for at least 2 hr to prevent reflux.

Medications

—Monitor and Teach Importance of Appropriate Medication

* Don't overmedicate with antacids: Over-the-counter antacids should not be taken more than one month without contacting physician.
* Assess ingredients of antacids to determine side effects and impact on nutritional status. Some antacids can increase body sodium, effect absorption of other medications, and cause decrease absorption of nutrients.

The Intestine

Diarrhea and Constipation All problems associated with the intestine involve treatment and/or prevention of diarrhea and constipation. Additionally, patients with other impairments experience difficulties with both these problems from time to time, and it is important to plan interventions that deal with the presenting or potential problem.

Interventions Specific to Diarrhea and Constipation

—*Assess and Teach Patient Importance of Determining Cause of Problem*

- Teach patient the definition of diarrhea and constipation so it can be determined first if the patient has a *real* problem rather than a perceived one of not defecating at the times they think they should. A change in usual pattern is more significant than a lifelong pattern that is unusual. Only by establishing this fact can it be determined that future intervention is necessary.

  Diarrhea—Abnormally frequent evacuation of watery stools.

  Constipation—Abnormally infrequent or difficult evacuation of hard, dry feces.

- Thoroughly assess the cause of diarrhea or constipation. Assess related symptoms such as pain, nausea, vomiting, bowel sounds, abdominal and rebound tenderness, the onset, and frequency of the problem. Explore possible side effects and interaction of medications.
- Teach patient how to monitor for color, frequency, consistency and pattern of symptoms.
- Teach assessment of food intake as indicator of possible cause of problem. (See "Chart of Foods" in Appendix I linked to intestinal problems.)
- Teach that home remedies or over-the-counter medications are not always indicated. Patients who are bombarded by television, radio, and magazine commercials often take nonprescribed medications when contact with the physician is the appropriate intervention.

- In both diarrhea and constipation increase fluid intake.
- **Remember,** there is no one way to treat diarrhea or constipation. The treatment is always determined by the cause.

—Teach Bowel Training and Regimes

Implications for bowel training include: decreased or limited mobility, dietary changes, depression, dehydration, anxiety, obstruction, and medications. Specific medications that can cause constipation include: antacids, analgesics, hypotensive agents, anticholingergics, iron preparations, opiates, anticonvulsants, and antidepressants. Suggestions for prevention of constipation are:

- Defecate when they first feel the urge and have a regular time of the day for evacuation.
- Position themselves so a sharp angle between the torso and the hips is achieved, that is, lean forward or sit with feet on a small stool.
- Increase activity and intake of fluids of at least 64 oz. a day.
- Hot fluids first thing in morning is often helpful.
- See "Nutrition—Diet" section, page 158.

Suggested Bowel Regime to Prevent Constipation (Physician orders necessary)

1. If simple interventions have not been successful, begin with a stool softener and gentle laxative:
   - Peri-Colace—1 capsule PO TID or
   - Senokot—2 tablets HS and 2 tablets BID or
   - Colace—1 capsule TID plus Dulcolax 5 mg PO or suppository HS

2. If no bowel movement in next 24 hours, add one of the following:
   - Senna or bisacodyl as described previously
   - Milk of Magnesia 30-60 mL PO HS (range: QD-BID)
   - Lactulose (Chronulac 10 g/15 mL) 30 mL PO HS (range: 15060 mL HS-BID)

3. If no bowel movement by 48 hours add one of the following:
   - Bisacodyl suppository, 10 mg PR
   - Magnesium citrate, 8 oz PO
   - Senna extract, 2.5 oz PO
   - Fleet enema

4. If no bowel movement by 72 hours perform rectal exam to rule out impaction.

   A. If *not* impacted, perform sequentially as needed:

      a. tap water enema
      b. soap suds enema
      c. milk and molasses enema
      d. oil retention enema

   B. If impacted:

      1. Check with M.D. for any cardiac arrythmia and/or disease before beginning to disimpact.
      2. Disimpact manually if stool is soft enough.
      3. Soften with glycerine suppository or oil retention enema, either disimpact manually at the time or plan a return visit later in the day or the next morning.
      4. Follow up with enema(s) until clear and then increase intensity of daily bowel prep.

Suggested Prophylactic Bowel Regime (Physician orders necessary)

When to Consider:

1. When the impaction has been resolved.
2. When analgesics or drugs known to cause constipation have been added to medication regime.
3. When patient becomes bedridden.

Drugs of Choice:

1. Colace: QD to TID
2. Surfak: 1 capsule QD to BID
3. Pericolace: 1 capsule QD to TID
4. Lactulose: 2 to 4 Tbsp. daily in divided doses.

Suggested Bowel Regime to Treat Some Forms of Diarrhea (Physician Orders Necessary)

Medication of Choice:

- Lomotil—1-2 tablets (maximum of 6 tablets in 24 hr)
- Imodium—1 q. 6 hr PRN
- Kaopectate—1-2 Tbsp. every 3-4 hr
- Metamucil—1 tsp. in 8 oz of water TID; absorbs the free fecal water

Nutrition—Diet to Prevent Constipation

- Increase significantly, if not contraindicated, the intake of fluids.
- Increase natural, weak-laxating foods such as prunes, apricots, and their juices, decaffeinated coffee, and tea as well as citrus fruits. Cooked and canned fruits and vegetables are lubricating also.
- Caffeine containing coffee and tea may stimulate gastrointestinal reflex, but they generally are constipating by increasing urine output and decreasing the fluid in the colon. Light tea is preferable to dark as it is low in caffeine and tannic acid which tends to "bind."
- Increase dietary bulk such as fresh fruits and vegetables, whole grain cereals, and bran. Wheat germ may be less irritating than bran if a patient has hemmorhoids (start with small amounts and gradually increase until effective).

Ulcerative Colitis and Crohn's Disease   Although these two diseases of the intestine are related in symptoms, each has different etiologies and prognosis:

- **Ulcerative colitis** is confined to the mucosal and submucosal layers of the wall of the colon and becomes diffuse involving the entire colon. The disease has a benign course over a long period of time and has frequent remissions.
- **Crohn's disease** affects all layers of the bowel and can occur in any area of the GI tract from the mouth to the anus. Crohn's Disease tends to start at a younger age than ulcerative colitis and symptoms are usually

progressive with no period of remission. Fistulae are the hallmark of Crohn's disease and are more common where there is involvement of the small bowel.

Interventions Specific to Ulcerative Colitis and Crohn's Disease

—*Teach Patient/Family to Monitor Symptoms*

- Assess difference between diarrhea and the constant loose stool associated with both diseases.
- Instruct on importance of frequent contact with physician to follow progression/remission of the disease.
- Reduce stresses in lifestyle so patient can decrease progression and symptoms of the disease.

Nutrition—Diet

- Patients with these complex and unpredictable diseases may constantly manipulate their diets in hopes of ameliorating symptoms.
- Active, long-standing disease can leave malabsorption problems due to gut scarring that results in declining nutritional status and a greater risk of infection.
- Patients with active disease need complete nutrition assessments on a routine basis to evaluate their status and provide guidelines for optimal nutrition.
- Patients often totally omit fruits and vegetables associated with cramping and diarrhea. Teach the importance of including mild-flavored, low-roughage fruits and vegetables in diet which are needed for natural lubrication and nutrients such as canned pears, applesauce, apricots, carrots, tender summer squash, winter squash, and potatoes.
- A difference of opinion exists on the inclusion of milk and dairy products. Often physicians order omission of all dairy foods while others omit only lactose-containing foods when patient has demonstrated a lactose intolerance on testing. If dairy products are omitted, nutritional supplementation for the calcium, protein, and other nutrients is implicated.

Diverticulitis and Diverticulosis

Diverticulosis is the presence of diverticula in the colon without inflammation. Diverticulitis is a complication of diverticulosis and is considered a form of inflammatory bowel disease that can have complications of peritonitis and abscess formation, fistulas, septicemia, obstruction, and hemorrhage.

Since many patients seen in the home experience diverticulosis in addition to other primary diseases, interventions center around prevention of diverticulitis as well as treatment of diverticulosis.

Interventions Specific to Diverticulitis and Diverticulosis

—*Teach Establishment of Bowel Regimen to Prevent Diverticulitis*

- Establish daily bowel routine and defecate when urge presents itself.
- Keep balance of exercise, nutrition, and fluids so constipation does not occur.
- Monitor consistency and pattern of stool. Patients can have loose stool all the time that is not considered diarrhea. This is not a concern because as long as some stool is moving through the colon, the probability of diverticulitis will be diminished.

—*Teach Plan of Action If Diverticulitis Occurs*

- Teach what normal stool looks like and how to differentiate, for example, blood, normal color, and changes that occur after ingestion of certain foods.
- Contact physician if constant, low crampy bowel pain occurs.
- Increase fluid intake to compensate for fluid loss through diarrhea.

Medication

- Since inflammatory bowel disease (diverticular disease, ulcerative colitis, and Crohn's disease) does not always respond to treatment and does not have a clear cause, new medications and treatment modalities will continuously be developed. Interventions center around understanding the goals and side effects of these treatments and medications on the specific patient.
- Antibiotics are often given and care should be taken to determine if presenting diarrhea is related to the antibiotic or the disease. Consult with the physician to determine if a change in antibiotic could be the most appropriate treatment for the diarrhea.

Nutrition—Diet

—*Teach Diet Plan for Both Prevention and Treatment of Diverticulitis*

- Current therapy suggests use of a high-fiber diet for diverticulosis omitting seeds and nuts which might become lodged in pouches. Avoidance of rough fibers is included for exacerbations of diverticulitis.
- Patients may manipulate their intake of fibrous foods to prevent painful upsets and will develop poorly balanced diets. If entire groups of foods are omitted, refer to a dietitian for evaluation and nutrition education.
- Test which spices are problematic and decrease amount of these spices used in cooking and seasoning.
- Decrease fatty food intake, but do not cut out all fats as they are needed for sound nutrition.
- Decrease crispy, fried foods which may present mechanical irritation to the intestine.

Bowel Resection

Most bowel resections are done for cancer, genetic problems, or traumatic injury. To plan interventions, it is essential to know what part and how much of the bowel was removed as this has a major impact on the treatment, assessment, and interventions developed for the patient. The following areas outline the intervention areas most specific to patients following a bowel resection of the small and large bowel.

Resection of the Small Bowel

—Teach Patient/Family Expectations Regarding Bowel Patterns

- Teach ways of handling diarrhea protection at home and in public. Commercial protectors for clothing are available.
- Reinforce teaching of short bowel syndrome outlining physiology related to removal of this part of bowel. Since the small bowel is responsible for absorption of nutrients, its removal raises concerns about nutrition.

Resection of the Large Bowel

—Teach Patient/Family Expectations Regarding Bowel Patterns

- Since the large bowel is responsible for absorption of fluids in the colon, loose pasty stool will become a normal pattern for the rest of the patient's life.
- If all the large bowel was removed, it will take at least one year after the surgery for the small bowel to adjust to the need to reabsorb fluids.
- If these patients experience stools that are more formed, assessment should determine if there has been a decrease in fluid intake, side effect of medications, or inaccurate dosage of Lomotil. Appropriate interventions can then be planned for these problems.
- As more surgical procedures are developed to prevent stomas such as "pull through" procedures, it is important to refer to an enterostomal therapist for up-to-date treatment.

Ostomy Care

—*Teach Way to Observe for a Healthy Stoma*

- A good stoma protrudes 0.25 to 0.5 in. and is 1 in. in diameter.
- There should be at least 2 in. of smooth skin around stoma, free of excoriation to hold appliance in place.
- It should be clearly visible to the patient.
- The stoma should be pink, the color of the mucous membrane of the mouth.
- All ostomy appliances should be changed at least every seven (7) days.
- To help patient adjust, refer to area as patient's stoma, avoid anyone giving it other names.

—*Observe and Teach Patient to Observe for Signs of Peristomal Irritation*

Signs and Symptoms

- **Incorrect Fitting of the Appliance.** Patients with new stomas need to be measured for proper fitting at least once a month for the first six months. If a patient loses or gains weight, remeasure stoma.
- **Stomal Laceration.** Results from shearing forces from a faceplate that is not properly bound to skin or cut properly to allow for a 1/16 to 1/8 in. of peristomal skin around stoma. If cut is severe, it will require surgical revision.
- **Slight Bleeding.** Bleeding from intestinal mucosa during appliance changes is very common and can be caused by slight injury to fragile tissue. Bleeding originating from within stoma can be potentially serious and always requires referral to physician.
- **Skin Excoriation.** Abrasion of the epidermis characterized by erythematous, weeping, bleeding areas and may be accompanied by pain due to loss of epidermis.

- **Skin Stripping.** Major problem with patients who remove appliance every day to irrigate or have frequent leaking problems. A skin barrier should be used to prevent stripping (*see* Appendix M for list of skin barriers). Some patients have allergic reactions to skin barriers or tape and should test materials before using. The incidence of allergy to barriers is low; many tapes are now hypoallergenic.
- **Epidermal Hyperplasia—Pseudo-Epitheliomatous Hyperplasia.** Characterized by thickened, wartlike skin, whitish raised area around stoma which is caused by too large opening of faceplate thus making the skin exposed to urine or discharge. Easily corrected by proper fitting of appliance.
- **Folliculitis.** Erythema at base of hair follicles brought about by using aggressive adhesives that tear hair from follicle and result in irritation or infection. Treatment: keep hair short by using an electric razor, not the blade type. To help remove tape, use water on edge of finger rather than using expensive, chemical solvents.
- **Urinary Crystal Formulation.** Caused by alkaline urine with pH greater than 7.0. Treatment: Keep urine acidic by using vitamin C and increase fluid intake.
- **Monilia.** Found around stoma and sometime in groin or under breast. Characteristics: tiny red spots, beefy red spots sometimes have white tops. Treatment: Cortiosteroids spray and anticandidal powder. Remove pouch, apply spray or powder once a day before replacing pouch. Any treatment needs prescription from physician.

—*Observe and Teach Problems That Interfere with Stomal Functioning*

- **Retraction** of stoma below the skin surface may be caused by scarring, surgical scars, and/or obesity which makes it difficult to keep appliance on. Greater convexity should be considered by use of a convex ring.
- **Prolapse** is an excessive protrusion of stoma due to

surgical difficulties or weakened abdominal muscles. Be sure type of pouch is large enough to encompass stoma. Use ostomy binder for support; sometimes surgical revision is necessary for permanent correction.

- **Necrosis** is caused by deficient blood supply. Stoma will get dark, dusky color. Results from ischemia which causes scarring and ultimately stomal retraction. Surgical revision is necessary.
- **Stenosis** occurs when opening becomes progressively smaller, thus resulting in a reduction of the flow. Stenosis is due to scarring at the skin and fascia levels because of repeated stomal dilations or disease processes. Treatment: dilation and surgical revision of stoma.
- **Peristomal hernias** are the bulging area around stoma caused by weakening abdominal muscles or fascial defects. Usually creates a management problem leading to leaking and skin irritation. An osto binder may be used or surgical intervention is often necessary.
- **Bowel obstruction, ileostomy dysfunction, food blockage** symptoms are the same as bowel obstruction. Caused by tumors, stricture of bowel, adhesive bands, inflammatory bowel disease, scarring process, or can be caused by eating high-fibrous foods, such as celery, chinese vegetables, even cantaloupe. Instruct patient to avoid high-cellulose foods and to chew all foods well. If food blockage is cause, lavage must only be done by physician or enterostomal therapist. Surgery may be indicated in obstruction.

Nutrition–Diet

- Teach importance of establishing a normal diet pattern. When patients experience loose stools due to poor water absorption, they often omit fibrous foods or decrease their fluid intake.
- If the remaining colon is not scarred and inflamed, lactic acid bacteria may be reintroduced by eating small amounts of yogurt or milk that contains active cultures of Lactobacillis. However, if the patient has been de-

termined to be lactose intolerant, the condition is likely
to remain after the surgery and the bacteria should not
be given.

- With bowel disease, there tends to be occasional intolerance to foods that contain higher than normal
spoilage bacteria, molds, or yeasts. Symptoms of persistent gas, bloating, and cramping are present. The
use of only freshly prepared foods, avoiding "leftovers" held in the refrigerator several days after cooking, is often helpful in eliminating these symptoms.

—Teach Importance of Adequate Hydration

- Force fluids since these patients are always dehydrated at least 10%, maybe even more during the first
year after the procedure.
- Teach patient kinds of fluids needed to maintain fluid/
electrolyte balance, such as, Gatorade, tea, broth, and
ways to prepare such as in popsicles, by mixing gelatin
with Gatorade, and such.

The Patient with Impairments of the Urinary Tract

Introduction

The urinary problem experienced frequently by home
care patients is urinary incontinence, often resulting in
the need for a long-term indwelling catheter. This section
will focus on this patient exclusively.

Types of Urinary Incontinence

- **Stress:** Occurs with physical exertion such as coughing, sneezing, and running.

- **Urgency:** Due to severe inflammation of the lower urinary tract and often in diabetes.
- **Overflow or Paradoxical:** Occurs in patients with totally decompensated bladders whose urine dribbles constantly.
- **Sphincteric Damage:** In patients with traumatic or surgical injury to the urinary sphincter.
- **Neurogenic:** Acquired or congenital which affects the neurologic components of the sphincteric mechanism.
- **Enuresis:** Involuntary loss of urine at night.

Causes

The most common causes of incontinence are:

- urinary tract infections
- defects present at birth
- damage to the nervous system
- diseases and injuries that directly or indirectly affect the urinary sphincter area
- loss of control that may come with aging

Treatment

- In some cases, the condition causing the problem can be corrected either by surgery or drugs.
- Bladder training and exercises are helpful with some types of incontinence.
- Specially designed devices have been developed that can assist the patient in coping if a cure is unavailable.
- Long-term indwelling catheters may need to be used to keep the patient comfortable and reduce deterioration of skin.

Interventions Specific for Incontinence

Interventions for the patient with incontinence involve several general areas that follow. Specific suggestions are made also for the care of the patient with an indwelling cathether.

—*Teach Ways to Preserve Renal Function and Prevent Urinary Track Infection*

- Teach importance of adequate hydration—fluids should be forced to 2.5 quarts/day (2.37 L) unless restricted for another reason.
- Keeping urine acid can assist in minimizing various problems related to skin, infection, odor, and formation of crystals. Ascorbic acid (vitamin C) 2 gm per day or more as prescribed alone or with Mandelamine divided over doses given every 4 hours around the clock and increasing fluids including cranberry juice have been found to decrease pH of urine and be the easiest, most successful way of keeping the urine acid. Be careful using cranberry juice if calories are a problem.
- Be sure patient empties bladder at least every 2 hours.

—*Teach Techniques for Preserving Skin Integrity*

- Provide special care to buttocks, groin, and perineal area.
- Keep skin clean and dry.
- A protective covering can be sprayed or wiped on the skin. (See Appendix M for list of skin sealants and barriers.)
- Teach available products for padding patient to collect urine and keep it away from skin. There are many new products on the market that can be used to allow the person to be ambulatory and decrease the odor associated with the traditional diapers.

—*Instruct in Bladder Training Techniques*

- Communicate clearly with both patient and family normal bladder function and reason for problem as well as how the program will work.
- Assess current bladder habits, that is, how often, at

what time, and under what circumstances voiding occurs.

- Develop a regulated fluid intake plan, limiting fluids before bedtime and when patient is going out of the home. Be sure to encourage fluids as these patients tend to decrease intake to prevent accidental incontinence.
- Develop a fixed schedule to develop the habit of voiding on schedule rather than on demand.

—*Teach Ways of Coping with Incontinence in ADLs*

- Assist patient in discussing feelings about problem and learning that methods are available to allow as normal a life as possible.
- Instruct on appropriate times to take diuretics to prevent nocturia and to accommodate when patient must leave home.
- Teach use of catheters if bladder training and padding techniques have not been successful.

—*Teach Use of External Catheter (Male)*

- External catheters have improved greatly in the past few years allowing patients to be more mobile. The McGuire urinal is washable and lasts about 6 months. Often patients who have a dribbling problem can use a penile clamp that is released every hour thus making lifestyle adjustments minimal.
- Teach careful technique and follow product directions when applying and disconnecting the device.
- Teach importance of assuring adequate circulation when the device is in use.
- Teach aseptic technique and appropriate schedule for use of device to prevent skin irritation.
- Teach care of leg bag—empty at frequent intervals, clean with solution of 1 quart water and 1 tablespoon bleach and dry thoroughly.
- Monitor color, clarity, and amount of urine produced daily.

—Teach Procedures for Indwelling Catheter (Female and Male)

- Observe urine for mucous, crystals, or sediment in drainage tube and on tip of catheter when removed.
- Keep record of condition of tip and stability of balloon when catheter is changed. This will assist in determining with the physician how frequently the catheter needs to be changed. There are no set times suggested for changing a long-term indwelling catheter; it is all determined by the individual patient situation.
- Conduct ongoing discussion with physician on the catheter's use and frequency of change.
- Teach perineal care. Wash around catheter area with mild soap and water frequently; no other preparation or medication need be applied.
- Assure cathether is attached to straight drainage or leg bag with bag emptied and cleaned frequently. Clean with solution of 1 quart water to 1 tablespoon bleach.
- Encourage patient to force fluids.
- Discourage catheter irrigations—these are usually the exception, not the rule.

—Teach Care of Ostomy, If Present

See Ostomy interventions in The Patient with Impaired GI Track Functioning, page 163.

The Patient with Impaired Skin Integrity

Introduction

The two most common impairments of skin integrity found in home care patients are pressure ulcers and surgical wounds. Interventions with the pressure ulcer, otherwise known as decubitus ulcer, bed sore, and pressure sore, center around either preventing or treating the problem. Care of pressure ulcers and surgical wounds involve interventions aimed at preventing infection and facilitating the healing process. This section will cover prevention of pressure ulcers and treatment of wounds which include both pressure ulcers and surgical wounds.

Interventions for Prevention of Pressure Ulcers

—*Teach Patient/Family the Causes of Ulcers*

- **Mechanical Forces Against the Skin:** bony prominence; objects such as mattress, chairs; interference with circulation; shearing force (bed raised over 30 degrees); friction; wrinkles and crumbs in bed linen.
- **Environmental Factors:** moisture; heat; drainage; dryness.
- **Physiological Factors:** weight; incontinence; immobility; infection; disease; age; skin condition; general nutrition; dehydration; poor circulation; sensory loss.

—*Monitor and Teach Patient/Family Ways to Remove or Modify Causes*

- Position Changes: ROM exercises, encouraging patient to move or if patient unable, moving patient (*see* page 214).
- Distribution of weight through use of flotation devices.
- Reduce Shearing: adjust bed position and change patient position.
- Reduce Friction: use pull sheets; put corn starch or powder on bottom sheet; sheepskin; keep bed clean, dry, and free of wrinkles; pad bed pan.
- Teach family to observe for reddened skin breaks over bony prominences.
- Provide Good Skin Care: use lotion, mineral oil, or petroleum jelly; massage bony prominences; keep skin dry and clean; control incontinence. (See page 167, Interventions for Incontinence.)

Interventions for Treatment of Wounds

Table 3.5 is helpful in recognizing and recording the progression of wounds.

Table 3.5. Wounds—Classification and Treatment

Classification	Signs and Symptoms*
Wounds Having Unbroken Epidermis	
No loss or interuption of intact epidermis, drainage not present	Erythema, edema, induration, pain, on touch, blisters, increased sheen
Partial Thickness Wounds	
Loss or interuption of intact epidermis, abrasion, minimal bleeding, granulation tissue present, epithelium at wound margins, drainage.	Erythema, edema, bleeding, exudate, scab, eschar and/or necrotic tissue, drainage, granulation, epithelial migration, induration, broken blisters

Classification	**Signs and Symptoms***

Full Thickness Wounds

Epidermis and dermis cleanly severed vertically; epidermal and dermal penetration opened; epidermis and dermis totally eroded; base of wound necrotic; granulation tissue may be present.

Erythema, periwound tissue warmth, edema, bleeding, pus, eschar and/or necrotic tissue, grainage, odor, granulation, epithelial migration.

Wounds with Deep Tissue Destruction

Epidermis and dermis divided with exposed fat and muscle or fascia. Epidermis and dermis totally eroded and/or lost. Underlying tissue involvement, delayed closure or dehiscence, base of wound necrotic epithelium at wound margins.

Erythema, edema, inflammation, bleeding, pus, eschar and/or necrotic tissue, drainage, exposed bone and tendon, granulation may be present, epithelial migration, odor.

Draining Wounds and Fistulas

Epidermis, dermis, and underlying tissue divided with some tissue loss; opening through the skin or wound is a conduit for drainage; epithelium at wound margins.

Erythema, edema, inflammation, odor, drainage, peri-fistula skin irritation.

---

*Not all symptoms are present in all cases.

—*Assess and Monitor Progression of Wound*

The most important method for determining the status of a wound is by simple physical examination. The following areas should be assessed and described fully in all recordings relative to status of the wound:

1. Location.
2. Size. Measure circumference in centimeters and whether partial or full thickness.
3. Location of epithelium, granulation, and necrosis.
4. Color, odor, texture, and approximate amount of drainage.

5. Condition of skin surrounding the wound and the edges of the wound.
6. Current or previously used treatments and their result.
7. Amount of time the wound has been known to exist.
8. Change in treatment and the results.

—*Provide and Teach Treatment of Wounds*

The treatment of wounds depends upon the type and condition of the wound and the treatment ordered by the physician. The following is a guideline of the most commonly used treatments linked to the stages of wounds. Policy and procedure of the agency as well as local preferences for treatment should also be considered.

Treatment for *All* Wounds

- Frequently assess skin and evaluate treatment—at least once a week.
- When choosing treatment, consider time, cost, and ease of application.
- Organize procedure and supplies so there is consistent application of dressing and other treatments of wound.
- Consider special equipment such as air mattress, acrilon pad, heel/elbow protectors, foam and bed cradle (see page 247).
- Remove the source of irritation (interventions are same as those listed for prevention of pressure ulcers on page 171).
- Continue to remove necrotic tissue to keep tissue area healthy and healing.
- Eradicate/prevent infection: Maintain aseptic technique; to date there is no evidence that antibiotics, either systemically or topically administered, can cleanse a contaminated wound. The partial thickness wound is rarely in danger of infection.
- Protect healthy tissue and keep wound appropriately hydrated. This is determined by the result desired from the dressing chosen.

—*Provide and Teach Dressing Technique*

- Teach reason, goals, and what to expect when dressing is changed. It is important to understand the ultimate objective of the dressing before applying it. The basic dressing has the following layers:

  1. Contact Layer—in direct contact with the wound.
  2. Absorption Layer—used to absorb any discharge.
  3. Cover Layer—used to stablize and anchor the first two layers.

- Teach procedure, stressing aseptic technique, and proper disposal of soiled dressings.
- Teach how to assess changes and progress of wound.
- Frequently communicate with physician and do not change procedure without an order.
- Teach family and observe technique/compliance. Ultimate role of home care is skilled teaching and ongoing observation of wound/skin.
- Table 3.6 will assist in evaluating various dressing techniques.

Table 3.6. Assessing Dressing Techniques

Technique	Pros	Cons
Dry→Dry	Good mechanical debridement. Absorption of nonviscous exudate.	Pain on removal. Possible detachment of viable epidermal surface cells on removal. Possible wound desiccation.
Wet→Dry	Good mechanical debridement. Good dilution and absorption of viscous exudate. Can be used in conjunction with medications in solution.	Pain on removal. Possible detachment of viable epidermal surface cells on removal.

(Continued)

Table 3.6—Continued

Technique	Pros	Cons
	Wound desiccation less likely than with dry→dry.	
Wet→Damp	Can be used in conjunction with medications in solution. Wound desiccation unlikely. Less pain on removal. Good dilution of viscous exudate.	Less effective debridement. Less absorptive property than dry dressing. Possible maceration of viable tissue. Increased possibility of bacterial proliferation. Little to no absorptive properties.
Wet→Wet	Least painful. Can be used in conjunction with medication in solution. Continuous cleansing of wound surface with dilution of exudate. No wound desiccation.	Less effective mechanical debridement. Possible maceration of viable tissue. Increased possibility of bacterial proliferation. Little to no absorptive properties.
Biologic Skin Substitutes	Little pain on removal. Most "natural" cover available for open wounds. Rapid liquefaction of necrotic debris.	Requires close monitoring of local response to "infection." Requires special storage. Time-consuming application.
Topical	Rapid eschar separation.	Requires close monitoring of local response to "infection."

Table 3.6—Continued

Technique	Pros	Cons
		Ointment base difficult to remove from tissue.
Hydrophilic Beads, gels, powders	Good absorption of exudate.	Cannot be used on "dry" wounds.
Synthetic	Rapid liquefaction of necrotic debris. Little pain on removal.	Requires close monitoring of local response to infection.

Reprinted with permission from the *American Journal of Nursing*, February, Volume 85, Number 2, "Artful Solutions to Chronic Problems," Janice A. Cuzzell. Copyright, 1985, American Journal of Nursing Company.

Nutrition—Diet

- In patients who have great metabolic demands, severe trauma, and/or interruption of healing due to infection, nutrition therapy should be aggressive, focusing upon adequate calories and protein for healing.
- Proteins should exceed 75 grams for patients with difficult wound healing and should come from biological sources such as eggs, milk, meat, fish, and poultry rather than supplements.
- Nutritional supplements (*see* Appendix J) may be needed if the patient is not eating well. They should be used following a meal, as an in between meal snack or as a late night snack so meal time consumption is not decreased.

The Patient with Cancer

Introduction

Cancer affects all body systems with resultant symptoms specific to that system. Additionally, the treatment and progress of the disease can affect other body systems and cause related problems.

Prior sections of this chapter addressed problems occurring in the various systems, this section will outline interventions related to the treatment of cancer—radiation, chemotherapy, oncologic emergencies, and pain management.

These guidelines must be used in relationship to the patient's other presenting problems so a comphrensive care plan can be developed.

Patients requiring home care for cancer fall in the following stages:

1. **Early Stage**—under treatment for newly diagnosed disease.
2. **Oncological Emergencies**—symptoms to watch for on long-term patients.
3. **Advanced Disease**—Those patients at the preterminal stage.

Interventions for All Cancer Patients

—Teach Patient/Family Information About the Disease

- More people are being cured today than ever before; estimates indicate 50% of all patients with serious forms of cancer will be long-term survivors.
- Survival rates for thyroid, endometrial, testicular, bladder, prostate, uterine, cervical, breast, Hodgkin's and laryngeal cancer are increasing dramatically.

- Clarify any misconceptions or prior experience with disease.
- Often patients know people who had cancer and are haunted by specifics of that person's disease thinking their treatment, pain, or death will be the same.
- Teach there is not just one drug or treatment for a specific cancer.

—*Allow Patient/Family to Verbalize Feelings About Disease*

- Assist patient in moving through the stages of reaction to disease outlined by Kubler Ross—denial, bargaining, anger, depression, and acceptance. People move between stages at varying times and often don't move through all stages.
- Encourage mutual support groups, counseling if indicated, and open communication between patient, family, and all health care providers. If appropriate, refer to hospice and other groups relative to specific forms of cancer.

—*Monitor and Teach Reactions of Treatment*

Treatment for cancer usually involves:

1. **Surgery and Possibility of Radiation**—for limited disease.
2. **Chemotherapy**—for systemic disease.
3. **Chemotherapy and/or Antibiotics**—for preterminal disease.

Interventions for Side Effects of Treatment

Surgery

Surgery involves the site(s) of the disease relative to a body system and has been discussed in previous sections. Plans of treatment should reflect the specific areas relevant to patient and surgical site.

Radiation

The extent of side effects in radiation varies from none to severe depending on the intensity and location of treatment and the condition and tolerance of the patient. Table 3.7 can be helpful in teaching patients what to expect from radiation therapy.

Table 3.7. Patient Instructions for Radiation Treatment

Possible Side Effects	Things Patients Should Know
All Sites	
Ink marks on skin where treatment is being given	Don't wash off the ink marks; they must stay on during course of Rx.
Dry or itchy skin; redness, tanning, sunburned look; may turn darker than usual	Don't wash area with soap or put on salves, deodorants, powders, etc., during or for 3 weeks after Rx.
	Keep treated areas out of sun. For future, use sunscreen at all times in sun.
	Do not apply hot or cold to skin.
	Do not rub, scrub, or scratch Rx area.
	If skin blisters, cracks or becomes moist, tell physician. Usually temporary and will disappear a few weeks after Rx is stopped.
Hair loss	Depends upon site of radiation; Areas affected—scalp, beard, eyebrows, armpits, pubic, and body hair. Usually grows back after 3 months; may be thinner and of a different color.
Extreme fatigue; a weak or tired feeling	Natural reaction and most common.

Possible Side Effects	Things Patients Should Know
	Extra rest periods and time of sleep required.
Loss of appetite	*See* eating hints in this section.
	Use Nutritional Supplements.
Sluggish bowels	*See* Constipation section.

Radiation to Head; Neck; Upper Chest; Mouth; Throat

Possible Side Effects	Things Patients Should Know
Sore throat, red tongue, white spots in mouth, sore mouth	Begins 2–3 weeks after Rx starts, decrease after 5th week, and ends 4–6 weeks after Rx.
Thick Saliva	Occurs during 3rd or 4th week of Rx.
	Rinse with club soda to thin out saliva. Use artifical saliva.
	See Mouth Care section, page 152.
Dry mouth	Occurs near end of Rx—lasts from several months to several years.
	See Mouth Care section, page 152.
Loss of taste or change in taste	Occurs during 3rd or 4th week of Rx, returns to normal from 3 weeks to 3 months after Rx completed; some taste buds may have been destroyed. May prefer egg and dairy dishes instead of meat.
Teeth problems	Have a complete dental exam before starting radiation.
	Brush teeth after each meal with baking soda and soft toothbrush. Don't use toothpaste.

(Continued)

Table 3.7—Continued

Possible Side Effects	Things Patients Should Know
	Radiation Rx can increase chances of getting cavities. Fluoride Rx may be ordered.
Earaches	Rx to brain can result in hardening of cerumen and impaired hearing; ear drops may be needed.
Drooping or swelling of skin under chin	Fatty tissue under chin shrinks after Rx. If lumps or knots on side of neck are noted, contact physician.
Loss of hair	Whiskers, sideburns, chest hair may disappear temporarily or permanently depending on dose and area. Rx to brain sometimes causes hair loss, usually temporarily. A hairpiece or wig can be used.

Radiation to Breast

Dry, tender, moist or itchy skin in armpit or under breast	Occurs during 3rd or 4th week of Rx. If itchiness persists, a commercial breast spray can be helpful, or area should be left open to air.
	A yellowish discharge can appear 2–3 weeks after Rx is completed.
	Sometimes the side effects of Rx continue for 4–6 weeks with skin reactions getting worse 2–3 weeks after completion of Rx.
	Prosthesis should not be worn till at least one month after Rx has ended.

Table 3.7—Continued

Possible Side Effects	Things Patients Should Know
Radiation to Upper Abdomen	
Nausea, vomiting, feeling of fullness	Suggest small meals, cool foods, decrease consumption of dairy products, cut out fatty foods.
Radiation to Lower Abdomen	
Diarrhea	Usually occurs during 4th week of Rx. Varies from 1–2 soft stools a day to as many as 10 watery stools a day.
Nausea, cramps, rectal burning with bowel movements (rare)	Start low-fiber diet early in Rx and follow physician's orders re: treatment for diarrhea.

Reprinted from "CHOICES Realistic Alternative in Cancer Treatment" by Marion Morra and Eve Potts. Copyright © 1979 by Marion Morra and Eve Potts. Reprinted by permission of Avon books, New York.

Nutrition–Diet

Nutrition Guidelines for Patients Experiencing Radiation to All Sites

- Modification and fortification of the diet should continue 4–6 weeks post-treatment to allow good tissue repair.
- N&V and anorexia must always be brought to the attention of the oncologist, as it may compromise Rx and/or deplete electrolytes.

Nutrition for Patients with Multimodal Treatments

- Breaks between therapies are best used to maximize nutrient intake.
- "Recall esophagitis" can occur when radiation-in-

duced esophagitis is treated with certain agents and
the patient experiences mucositis once again.
- Periodic nutritional assessment should be planned
  when patient on aggressive protocols. Problem areas
  in eating, digestion, and elimination can be discov-
  ered which the patient may have failed to report to
  the oncologist.

Nutrition for Patients with Radiation to Mouth, Throat, and Esophagus

- Warm to cold food is best tolerated.
- Food consistency should be modified to eliminate sticky
  or gummy foods and those that have sharp edges or
  particulate matter which cause irritation to tender mucosal membranes.
- Nonacid foods that are semi-solid or liquid are easily
  tolerated.
- Making foods with lubrication such as yogurt, sour
  cream, ice cream, gravies, and sauces aides in swallowing.
- Patients with reduced salivary output should have moist
  foods and artifical saliva if necessary.
- Patients who experience severe mucositis require use
  of local anesthetic before eating.

Nutrition for Patients with Radiation to Gastric and Bowel Areas

- A low-fiber diet should precede Rx to minimize irritation of mucosal linings and continue well past Rx
  to ensure restoration of tissue.
- A balanced, high-calorie, high-protein diet is used to
  counter malabsorption side effects.
- Nutritional supplements in liquid or pudding are extremely helpful. Patients often must be urged to try
  them for they think they are unpalatable or their condition is worsening. Available nutritional supplements and their properties are listed in Appendix J.
- Lactose intolerance is common if the small bowel is
  irradiated. Active cultures in both milk and yogurt or
  milk containing lactic acid bacteria may be slowly
  introduced after the Rx is completed.

Chemotherapy

Chemotherapy is the use of chemicals to destroy the cancer cells, either by interfering with their growth or by preventing them from reproducing. Important aspects of the care plan in these patients are:

—Teach Patient Importance of Keeping Up Schedule of Treatments

- Teach that to receive maximum benefit from Rx, medication must be given in regular doses as prescribed.
- Assist with transportation to treatments.

—Teach Interventions Specific to Type of Medication Used

See Table 3.8, page 186.

Observe for Signs and Symptoms of Infection

Patients who receive chemotherapy become granulocytopenic and are at high risk of developing infections. Since during therapy the patient has minimal white blood cells, defenses are down and the common symptoms of infection such as exudate, ulceration or fissure, local heat, swelling, and regional adenopathy are less present. Fever, erythema, and local pain or tenderness are the only reliable indicators of infection in these patients. The five most common localized infections and the symptoms seen in immunosuppressed patients are:

1. Pharyngitis: sore throat or mouth, and fever.
2. Skin infection: erythema, pain, and fever.
3. Anorectal infection: erythema, pain, and fever.
4. Urinary tract infection: fever is common while usual symptoms of UTI (dysuria, frequency, and urgency) occur less often.
5. Pneumonia: fever and infiltrate on chest x-ray, while usual symptoms of cough and purulent sputum rarely occur.

Table 3.8. Cancer Chemotherapuetic Agents

Drug	Mode of Action	Toxicities/ Complications	Nutritional Implications
Antimetabolites	Interfere with metabolism of essential amino acids	Bone marrow suppression, mucosal, and gut ulceration	Anorexia, malabsorption of Vitamin B_{12}, fat, and other nutrients.
6-Mercaptopurine 5-Fluorouracil Methotrexate			Diet as tolerated; do not schedule meals close to Rx. Vitamin restrictions, that is, folic acid.
Alkylating Agents Chlorambucil	Alkylation of DNA and RNA, causing fragmentation of chromosomes	Marrow suppression, mucosal, and gut ulceration, immunosuppression	During Rx: cold bland fluids, ice creams, milk shakes to prevent ulcers.
Cyclophosphamide Nitrogen Mustard		Hemorrhagic cystitis (cyclophosphamide)	Avoid: acidic foods, spices, hot foods. Increase fluids.
Antibiotics Doxorubicin chloride Daunorubicin	Reduces cellular reproduction by binding DNA to block RNA;	Bone marrow suppression, megaloblastic anemia, immuno-	Adequate hydration. Alkalization of urine. Vitamin B_{12} supplement.

Actinomycin Mithramycin	cell division is prevented.	suppression, uric acid production, anorexia.	High-nutritional-density snacks.
Hormones Androgen Estrogen Progesterone Corticosteroids	Large doses alter hormonal balance modifying growth of cancer cells susceptible to hormonal influence.	Immunosuppression, edema, hypertension, loss of calcium, potassium, nitrogen, anorexia/increased appetite.	Restrict sodium. Possible Rx with diuretic. Calcium and Potassium supplement.
Vinca Alkaloids Vinblastine Vincristine	Disorganize and destroy spindle causing mitotic arrest in cellular reproduction.	Marrow suppression, paresthesias, loss of DTRs, paresis, jaw and abdominal pain, constipation, uric acid production, anorexia, weight loss.	Adequate fluids high calories, high-protein diet with high-density nutrient supplements. Flexible meal times.
Asparaginase	Asparagine deficiency, inhibits protein synthesis	Chills, fever, liver dysfunction, immunosuppression, pancreatitis. Drowsiness and uncontrolled body movements can continue several weeks after last dose.	Low-protein diet. Increase fluids.

Other symptoms to observe:

- Watch for subtle signs of infection such as any unusual sensation like an itch or flutter.
- Observe behavioral changes, especially when not manifesting a fever.

—Teach Measures to Prevent Infection in Cancer Patients

Preventing infection in the immunosuppressed patient centers around maximizing the patient's defense and decreasing the exposure to potential pathogens. Infection is the cause of death in about 60% of patients with leukemia, 65% of patients with lymphoma, and 40% of patients with solid tumor.

The following measures should be selectively implemented with ongoing discussion with the physician and monitoring of blood tests to determine the level of precautions needed:

- Maintain skin/mucosa integrity as it is the first line of defense against bacterial and fungal infections. This is especially important in patients with leukemia, non-Hodgkin's lymphoma, radiation therapy, surgery, hyperalimentation, and solid tumors, both local and disseminated.
- Avoid crowds and exposure to infections, especially URI.
- Teach conservation techniques to reduce excessive physical stress (see page 209).
- Avoid injury to skin and mucous membranes (mouth care, skin lotion, bruises, and contusions).
- Avoid unnecessary urinary catheterization and intravenous cannulas.

On high risk patients; that is, those who have an absolute granulocyte count of 500 per mm or less, the following precautions should be implemented:

- Wash all fresh food well and peel skin if food is not cooked. Use of canned food may be recommended.

- Avoid raw eggs, pepper, yogurt, moldy cheeses, and salads.
- Use small containers of food and use contents completely at one serving to prevent leftovers.
- Patients should have their own eating utensils, dishes, and glasses.
- Avoid cut flowers and houseplants, water standing in containers for long periods is media for bacteria.

Nutrition—Diet

—Teach Nutritional Guidelines Related to Chemotherapy

- High-protein, high-calorie foods should be used with increased vitamin A and C to prevent infection.
- OTC vitamin supplements should always be cleared with physician to prevent interference with drug therapies.
- Mouth ulceration—soft, nonacid foods, usually warm or cold to minimize irritation.
- Drink with straw or substitute liquids for solids.
- N&V following Rx is short lived, minimize food intake for 1–2 days following Rx.
- Family should avoid use of aromatic foods which can increase patient's nausea.
- Patients with daily drug ingestion can have long-term eating problems if side effects are nausea, persistent taste aberrations, or intolerance of food aroma. Continuous sips of water, use of mildly flavored warm or cool foods, and use of hard candy, if allowed, are helpful.
- After cessation of Rx, good dietary habits should be continued to promote healing and restoration of body tissue.

Oncologic Emergencies

Oncologic emergencies are manifestations related to the pathophysiology and treatment of cancer that are life-threatening in nature. The potential for these emergencies requires constant assessment to identify patients at risk and to observe for early signs and symptoms of these manifestations. These emergenices present as a sudden change in the disease process and require immediate medical intervention.

Several oncologic emergencies have insidious onsets that can be first seen by the home care nurse. It is crucial that a differential diagnosis be made when working with a cancer patient in the home by taking into consideration the possibility of an oncologic emergency rather than attributing the problem to another cause or condition. The most common oncologic emergencies found in home care patients follow with definitions of those not commonly known.

1. Increased Intracranial Pressure.
2. Spinal Cord Compression occurs as a result of the presence of a neoplasm in the epidural space of the spinal cord. When the neoplasm fills the epidural space, direct compression of the spinal cord through an intact dura results.
3. Superior Vena Cava Syndrome (SVCS). The compression of the superior vena cava and its tributaries with subsequent engorgement of the vessels of the upper trunk.
4. Bowel Obstruction.
5. Hypercalcemia. An elevation in the serum calcium level above the normal level of 9 to 11 mg/100 mL.
6. Syndrome of Inappropriate AntiDiuretic Hormone (SIADH). A syndrome exhibited by elevated blood levels of the antidiuretic hormone (ADH), retention of water (water intoxication), and hyponatremia.
7. Sepsis.
8. Thrombosis.

    Table 3.9 can help in differentiating the possible oncologic emergencies as related to tumor type so then further assessment can be done.

Advanced Disease

Care of the patient with advanced stages of cancer often focuses on dealing with pain in addition to problems associated with the involved system and acceptance, family support, and grief and grieving.

—*Teach and Monitor Requirements and Reactions to Pain Medication*

Most cancers cause no pain in the early stages. Among those with advanced disease, more than half have little or no pain or discomfort. Since cancer pain has the unique characteristics of being both severe and of long duration, the approach to controlling pain can be varied. Many HHAs, hospices, and physicians have protocols for pain that should be followed.

Table 3.10 indicates the types of analgesics most used for pain control in cancer patients.

Table 3.9. Oncologic Emergencies Seen in the Home

Tumor Type	Increased Intracranial Pressure	Spinal Cord Compression	SVCS	Bowel Obstruction	Hypercalcemia	SIADH	Sepsis**	Thrombosis	Oncological Emergency
Bone*		X			X				Pathologic fracture
Bladder				X					Renal failure
Brain*	X								
Breast		X			X	X			
Colon/Rectum				X					
Esophagus			X		X				Hemorrhage
Kidney		X			X				Hemorrhage
Lung		X	X		X	X	X	X	Renal failure

							Hyperglycemia
Melanoma							
Ovary				X			
Pancreas	X			X	X	X	X
Prostate		X				X	X
Sarcoma							
Stomach							
Testes						X	
Thyroid							
Uterus				X			
Leukemia						X	
Lymphoma	X		X		X	X	
Myeloma	X		X				

SOURCE: Johnson, BL, and J Gross. *Handbook of Oncology Nursing* New York: John Wiley and Sons, 1985. Used with Permission.
*Risk for oncological emergency exists for patients with either primary amd metastatic disease in these sites.
**Risk for oncological emergency exists for any patient experiencing bone marrow suppression from chemotherapy or radiation therapy.

Table 3.10. Analgesics Used for Pain

	Drug	Dosage Forms	Duration (Hours)
MILD PAIN	Aspirin	Tabs: 325 mg Suppositories: 325 mg, 650 mg	4–6
	Acetami- nophen (Datril) (Tylenol)	Tabs: 325 mg, 500 mg Suppositories: 650 mg Liquid: 500 mg/15 mL	4–6
	IBUPROFEN (Nuprin) (Motrin)	Tabs: 300, 400, 600 mg	4–6
MODERATE PAIN	Codeine	*Tylenol #3* = 300 mg Tylenol and 30 mg (½ gr) Codeine *Tylenol #4* = 300 mg Tylenol and 60 mg (1 gr) Codeine	4–6
	Oxycodone	*Percocet* = 5 mg Oxycodone and 325 mg Acetaminophen base *Percodan* = 5 mg oxycodone and 325 mg aspirin base *Tylox* = 5 mg oxycodone and 500 mg acetaminophen-capsulated	4–5
SEVERE PAIN	Morphine	Oral Tabs: 15 mg, 30 mg Oral Solution: 10mg/5 mL 20mg/5 mL IV Drip titrated	4–5
	Hydro- morphone (Dilaudid)	Tabs: 1 mg, 2 mg, 3 mg, 4 mg Suppositories: 3 mg each	4–5
	Levorphanol (Levo- Dromeran)	Tabs: 2 mg Injectable	4–5
	Methadone (Dolo- phine)	Tabs: 5 mg and 10 mg	4–6
	Meperidine (Demerol)	Tabs: 50 mg and 100 mg	2–4

Control in the Cancer Patient

Half Life (Hours)	Equianalgesic Doses (mg)		Comments
	IM	Oral	
			Use with caution in patients with potential for bleeding. Enteric-coated forms available. Take with fluids or food to avoid gastric irritation.
			Reduced incidence of GI bleeding and irritation. Markedly reduced interactions with other protein-bound meds— Important consideration for chemotherapy patients.
			Give with meals/milk to reduce GI side effects. May take 2 weeks to realize optimum effect.
3−4	130	200	More constipating than other narcotics. Has antitussive effect. Potential drug dependency.
	15	30	Synthetic codeines used in combination. Contains all characteristics of addiction. Contains all characteristics of codeine, including allergenic response.
2−3	10	30−60	Drug of choice due to variety of convenient dosage forms and effectiveness, related to herion.
2−4	1.5	8	Onset of action as fast as injected morphine but in oral form.
	2	4	Morphine but in oral form.
22−25	10	20	May be difficult to titrate safely due to cumulative effect. Duration and half life increase with repeated use.
3−4	75	300	Not recommended due to short duration and poor oral absorption.

The Patient with Altered Cognitive Functioning

Introduction

Because of the increase in the aging population, home care nurses will be increasingly called upon to assess and treat elders with impaired cognitive functioning. While the primary presenting problem may be physiological, it is important to understand the impact impaired cognitive functioning has on the patient's ability to comprehend and follow treatment interventions. Conversely, the impact of an altered physiological state has an effect on the patient's cognitive functioning which must also be considered in planning interventions.

In advanced stages of Senile Dementia of the Alzheimer's Type (SDAT), the nurse may be asked to manage problems associated with urinary incontinence, decubiti, severe constipation, and eating difficulties.

The following interventions are meant to be guidelines for working with these patients and teaching families to manage the problems of dementia.

Specific Interventions

—Teach Family the Progression of the Disease

Senile Dementia of the Alzheimer's Type causes progressive decline in intellectual functioning. The progression usually follows this path:

1. Mild forgetfulness.
2. Difficulty finding words and names.
3. Decreased knowledge of recent events in their life (short term memory loss).
4. Increased difficulty in social settings, that is, shopping, visiting, and such.

5. Withdrawal from challenging situations.
6. Disorientation to time.
7. Memory loss for past events.
8. Increased difficulty and/or inability to perform ADLs.
9. Disorientation to place.
10. Memory loss for events in their past lives.
11. Inability to communicate.
12. Incontinence.

—Teach Family Assessment for Judgement, Orientation, and Memory Loss

Judgement

- In assessing judgement, consider if patient's decisions are appropriate to their needs and circumstances.
- Are they denying problems/needs resulting in self neglect?
- Evaluate judgement in many areas including dress, medication use, diet, locking of doors on house, use of stove, and so on.
- Patients often report they can perform ADL activities independently when they can't.

Orientation

People lose orientation in the following order:

1. First—Time
2. Second—Place
3. Third—Person

Find out if person can find the rooms in their house, then clothing, food, emergency exit, telephone, and specifics about any treatment regimes or medications.

With the person who lives alone, the family should question the patient frequently regarding the following areas:

- In case of an emergency, can the patient get out?
- Who would they call?
- Can they correctly give their name and location to the police and/or fire department?

Memory Loss

Normal progression of memory loss is:

1. Loss of memory for recent events.
2. Loss of memory for events from past.
3. Finally, loss of memory for events from remote past.

Memory loss may be inconsistent with recall of some items and not others, or patient may recall something at one time and be unable to recall it again at another time.

Instruct that recall of phone numbers of family and emergency numbers is important for safety. Many people cover memory deficits by being vague, evasive, or confabulating (making up appropriate responses). Family members should be especially aware of this to evaluate safety appropriately.

Gear Care to the Level of Cognitive Functioning

- When developing a care plan that involves a medical problem, always consider the level of cognitive functioning and gear teaching to this level.
- In the early to middle stages of deterioration, the patient can still do a great deal for himself. In this stage it is important to direct teaching to the patient as well as to the family.
- In the later stage of severe deterioration, teaching should be *only* to the family/caregiver. It is important at this stage to teach the family that there is no arrangement of the environment that can keep the patient oriented because the disease has damaged the brain cells. This is when the family needs support and respite.

—*Teach Patient and Family Structure as Key to Living*

Structure is important in helping the patient maintain a sense of mastery over the environment. Structure can be outlined in the following three categories:

1. Teaching

   - Give simple directions.

- Use nouns, not pronouns.
- Write everything down, including steps to a procedure, times for treatments, and phone numbers.
- Give one direction at a time and allow time for patient to respond.
- Set up check lists for treatments, exercises, medications, and any other routines that need to be monitored or directed.

2. Medications

- Prepour medications and use envelopes or pill boxes.
- Use color codes and check lists as needed.

3. Daily Routine

- Teach patient/family to establish a fairly standard schedule for meals, medications, treatments, and activities. This can help the patient be as independent as possible while also making him feel more secure.
- Family needs to plan supports so they can get out of house. Families often deny their own needs when providing 24 hour care.

—*Teach Family Importance of Ongoing Evaluation*

- If appropriate, the family can administer MSQ and any other testing necessary to monitor current mental status and any changes (*see* page 43).
- Any abrupt altered change in mental status needs thorough evaluation as there is usually an underlying physical cause. Assess concurrent diseases and prescribed medications.

—*Recognize Catastrophic Reactions*

A catastrophic reaction happens when a patient finds himself in situations that demand he perform tasks beyond his capabilities. He then feels overwhelmed and manifests this in a variety of ways, most usually in stubborness, angry outbursts, and/or negativism.

Teach the family to recognize these reactions and avoid trying to reason or argue with the patient during the reaction. The correct way to handle this situation is to remain calm, speak slowly, and to remove the person from the situation.

Reality Orientation

- Calendars and clocks should be used to keep the patient oriented to time.
- Label rooms, drawers, and other areas in house to help with orientation to place.
- In later stages of dementia, everyone who comes in contact with the patient should tell the patient their name and title to keep them oriented to person as much as possible.
- The patient should be called by their given name, not a nickname or titles, like Grandma, Dad, and such.
- Always tell the person exactly what you will be doing to avoid anxiety and to reinforce their memory.

—Refer to Other Agencies

Many self-help and mutual support groups have been developed for patients with Alzheimer's Disease and their families. Day care centers can be a useful resource to provide respite for families. Depending on other aspects of the patient and family situation, other community resources may be appropriate.

Medications

There is no medication available to treat dementia. Some have been and are being tried to increase cerebral circulation and memory. In experimental trials these medications have helped a few people but no significant changes or results have occurred. Medication is effective with the associated psychiatric symptoms of depression, agitation, anxiety, and psychosis manifest in hallucinations and delusions, as well as insomnia.

If a patient is being given medications for concurrent medical conditions the following should be part of the interventions specific to the patient with dementia:

- Taking medications as prescribed: These patients easily over- and underdose themselves.
- Watch for multiple medications with anticholinergic (beta blocker, antihistamines, antipsychotic meds) side effects. These may be cumulative and may cause altered mental state.
- Monitor drug interactions specific to the meds. Many drugs have side effects of confusion that are exaggerated in patients with dementia.
- Observe for signs of depression. Cardiac medications and antihypertensives may produce depression as a side effect.

Nutrition—Diet

- Maintain adequate nutrition. If the patient is not on a therapeutic diet they need a nutritionally sound basic diet.
- Maintain adequate hydration. With memory impairment, these patients may forget to eat and drink. In severe dementia frequent small feedings are useful.
- Teach special dietary tips. More active patients need high-calorie, not high-sugar foods and snacks; finger foods and small portions should be used; a decrease in caffeine intake as well as mechanical soft diet and nutritional supplements is helpful.
- Establish toileting schedules and high-fiber diets to prevent constipation.

4

Procedures

This chapter includes procedures commonly used by the nurse in the home. Procedures were chosen for this chapter because they are:

1. used frequently with home care patients;
2. modified for the home environment;
3. needed as quick reference guide in the home; and
4. applicable to patients with various diagnoses, therefore not lending themselves to an individual section in Chapter 3.

Additional guidelines are given in this chapter regarding the sterilization of equipment and solutions in the home. These are included so when these procedures are required on a long-term basis or when financial resources are limited, the patient will have access to the safest, most economical care possible.

Foot Care

1. Bathe feet daily with warm water and mild soap. Dry well between toes and apply skin cream.
2. Inspect feet daily for cuts or cracks and observe for signs of infection. If skin is broken, wash, pat dry, but do not rub. Apply hydrogen peroxide and wrap area with sterile gauze, careful not to place tape on skin. Encourage to seek care immediately for even simple problems.
3. Wear shoes and socks that fit well. Wrinkles and holes can cause areas of friction that create blisters or calluses.
4. Have corns and calluses trimmed at the doctor's of-

fice. Do not cut with a razor blade or use harsh products. Clip toenails straight across.

5. Always wear slippers with hard soles since bare feet
   invite injury, and feeling can be diminished in feet.
6. Never use hot water bottles or heating pads on feet
   or legs.
7. Avoid wearing anything tight around legs such as
   garters or stockings. Don't cross legs while sitting.
8. Do not smoke as nicotine decreases circulation.

Collecting Specimens

The nurse may be called upon to collect specimens for
laboratory tests while in the home. Although not a laboratory technician, it is possible for a nurse who is profi-
cient in venipunctures to be able to collect certain specimens in a correct manner so the laboratory can complete
the appropriate tests.

The following commonly used tests for blood, urine,
and feces are outlined as the basic information needed to
collect the specimen upon receipt of physician's orders.
Although laboratories have procedures and supplies specific to their practices, the following are commonly used
procedures, equipment, and instructions.

Basic Information

1. Check the specific test(s) ordered—call M.D. if necessary.
2. Have supply of appropriate containers for collection
   (see following list) as well as supplies for the venipuncture.
3. Clearly indicate the patient's full name and date collected on *every* specimen.
4. Store the specimen as directed, based on the test, and
   put in a safe place.
5. Be sure the lab knows where the results are suppose
   to be reported.
6. Plan the time of the collection to coincide with the
   ability to return it to the lab within a reasonable amount
   of time.

7. Don't expose specimens to extreme temperatures of the car for prolonged periods.

Specimen Containers for Collecting Blood

Speckled Top Tubes contain a gel that, when centrifuged, forms a layer between serum and packed red blood cells. They contain no anticoagulants and are used for various chemistries. If the test is also to determine glucose the blood should not be allowed to set more than 45 minutes since glycolysis will occur leading to low glucose values and an invalid result.

Lavender Top Tubes contain EDTA (an anticoagulant). Draw volume may be 2–10 mL. These tubes are used for tests performed on whole blood samples. Each tube should be inverted immediately at least 10 times to ensure adequate mixing of blood and anticoagulant.

Gray Top Tubes contain a glycolytic inhibitor. Draw volume may be 3–10 mL. These tubes are used most often for glucose determinations in serum or plasma samples. Invert at least 10 times to ensure adequate mixing of the blood and anticoagulant.

Blue Top Tubes contain sodium citrate and citric acid. Draw volume may be 2.7 or 4.5 mL. These tubes are used for coagulation studies requiring plasma samples. The tube should be filled to obtain a proper ratio of blood to anticoagulant and immediately inverted at least 10 times.

Green Top Tubes contain heparin. Draw volume may be 2–15 mL. These tubes are used for tests performed on plasma samples.

Commonly Ordered Urine Tests and Collection Directions

Routine Urinalysis and Urine Culture   A clean voided midstream specimen collected in a sterile cup is required.

MALE PATIENT   Thoroughly clean glans penis with antiseptic towelettes and collect cleanly voided midstream specimen in a plastic cup. Cover and refrigerate immediately.

FEMALE PATIENT   Spread the labia and cleanse the area using antiseptic towelettes. Cleanse on each side of the urinary meatus, then cleanse the meatus. While the labia are still held apart, a small amount of urine should be passed into the toilet and discarded; then a midstream specimen is collected in a container. Cover and refrigerate immediately.

Collection of 24-Hour Urine Specimen   Have the patient empty bladder at the beginning of the period and discard this urine. Collect all urine voided during the next 24 hours and store in a cool place. At the end of the 24-hour collecting period the bladder is emptied, and this urine is added to those already collected. Note that inadequate preservative, loss of any voided specimens, or the inclusion of two morning collections are problems often encountered in the collection of 24-hour urine specimens.

Commonly Ordered Parasitology Specimens and Directions for Collection

Feces should be collected directly in a clean wide-mouth container with a tight fitting lid. Bismuth, barium, oils, such as mineral oil, antacids, and various antibiotics render fecal specimens unsuitable for examination.

Formula for Calculating I.V. Flow Rates and Infusion Times

$$\frac{\text{Flow Rate}}{\text{(drops/min)}} = \frac{\text{Drops in 1 mL x total mL}}{\text{Total time (min)}}$$

$$\frac{\text{Infusion time}}{\text{(hour)}} = \frac{\text{Total volume to be delivered}}{\text{mL being delivered/hr}}$$

—*Hot Packs (May need physician order)*

Objectives

To increase blood flow to the area being treated and/or to relieve muscle spasm

Indications

- Trauma after first 36–48 hours.
- Subacute inflammatory condition, that is, arthritis, bursitis, periarthritis.
- Chronic inflammatory condition—ligament and tendon tears, chronic postural stress.
- Post fracture.
- Neuromuscular condition.
- In preparation for other treatment procedures, that is, massage, stretching traction.

Contraindications

- Over thick keloid formations where sensation is absent.
- On extremities if there is arterial insufficiency.
- On open wounds.

Duration of Treatment

30 minutes.

Variations

Heating pad, hot water bottle, hot pack, paraffin, hot water baths.

Cold Packs

Objectives

To relieve pain, reduce edema, reduce spasticity.

Indications

- Traumatic injuries and insect bites.
- Reduction in spasticity.
- Headaches.

Contraindications

- Hypersensitivity to cold.
- The very young or very old.

- PVD, acute heart conditions, hypertension.
- New incisions.

Duration of Treatment

20 minutes.

Variations

Ice pack or slush pack, which can be made of ⅓ alcohol and ⅔ water, placed in plastic bag and kept in freezer; or frozen wet towel kept in plastic bag, molded to size needed, and kept in the refrigerator.

Administering Eye Medication

Although the application of eye medication may seem easy, there are several points to remember when teaching patients and families to ensure the medication reaches the eye, and that injury does not occur. The steps in each procedure follow.

Eye Drops

1. The patient should sit with his head back or lie down on his back and turn his head toward the side of the affected eye so the medication can flow away from his tear duct.
2. It should be clear on the medication bottle the dose and which eye is to receive the medication. Remember:
   O.D. = Right Eye
   O.S. = Left Eye
   O.U. = Both Eyes
3. Always wash hands before giving medications.
4. Using forefinger, pull lower lid down gently to form a cul-de-sac and have the patient look upward.
5. Drop medication into center of lower lid and instruct the patient to close his eyes slowly and not to squeeze them.

Eye Ointment

Procedure is similiar to eye drops in that the ointment is applied gently along the inner lower lid. Be careful not to touch the eye with the end of the tube.

Energy Conservation Techniques

Patients with breathing problems or physical limitations must learn to pace themselves and learn new ways to save energy with minimal changes in their lifestyle. Teaching the following techniques and referral to an occupational and/or physical therapist for modifications in the home are helpful.

- To minimize the "burst of activity" demanded on the body when awaking, teach stretching and relaxing exercises to be done in bed before arising.
- Keep robe, slippers, socks, and underwear beside the bed so some dressing can be done sitting on the edge of the bed.
- When bathing, use a bath stool and a hand-held shower head as well as a terry robe which eliminates the energy needed to dry the body.
- Avoid elaborate hairdos that need setting and extended use of hand held blowers.
- Avoid the use of any aerosol sprays, except those prescribed by a physician.
- Avoid tight belts, bras, and girdles, and stick to loose clothing that doesn't restrict the chest and abdominal expansion. Use suspenders, slacks, slip-on-type shoes and socks rather than pantyhose to minimize the effort expended in dressing.
- For moving around the house, use a small rolling utility cart that has three shelves to carry things. On the cart a small stool or camping seat can be carried so bottom drawers or other low jobs will not require stooping but sitting.
- When carrying things upstairs, lift things on an exhale and put them down in two to three steps. Rest, and then pick them up again, exhaling each time.

- If the house has stairs, put a chair to sit on at the top or bottom of the stairs to use for a rest.
- Small or large tongs are helpful in picking up small items and items high on shelves.

Breathing Techniques

Breathing exercises strengthen respiratory muscles and decrease energy consumption. The technique of a deep inspiration followed by pursed lip expiration decreases the rate of breathing and promotes breathing in a coordinated pattern. Abdominal (diaphragmatic) breathing is practiced with pursed lip expiration. Breathing at a slower more efficient rate the work of breathing is decreased, and, thus, less energy is expended.

Relaxation Exercises

Relaxation is very important in obtaining good breathing control. Once the feeling of muscular tightness is recognized, it will be easy to recognize the contrast of muscular relaxation.

Remember:

- Practice daily.
- Perform these exercises in a quiet, comfortably warm room.
- Avoid pain.
- Perform all exercises slowly and smoothly.
- Breathe naturally throughout all exercises.

Shoulder Shrugging

Sit in a chair and let arms hang loosely by you side. Shrug your shoulders and tighten muscles as much as possible. Hold the position until you feel the muscles of the neck and shoulders are tight. Hold for a count of five. Release the tension, letting the shoulders drop. Repeat three times.

Head Circles

Sitting in a chair, let arms hang loosely, shoulders relaxed, and drooped. Roll head slowly and loosely from side to side. Reverse direction of head circle. Repeat three times to each side.

Shoulder Rolling

Sitting in a chair with arms resting at sides, clinch the right fist tightly and bend elbow. Hold for the count of five. Release the fist and contraction of the arm and allow the arm to straighten slowly. Repeat three times.

Arm and Fist Tightening

Lying on your back with arms resting at sides, clinch the right fist tightly and bend elbow. Hold for the count of five. Release the fist and contraction of the arm and allow the arm to straighten slowly. Repeat three times.

Arms Overhead with Chest Tightening

Lying on your back with arms resting at both sides, slowly raise extended arms overhead until palms of hands meet. Slowly press palms together until you feel a contraction of your chest muscles. Hold for a count of five. Gradually release the pressure at the hands and return arms to your side. Repeat three times.

Diaphragm Breathing

Objective   To use the diaphragm correctly to keep the lungs fully expanded to make breathing more efficient and prevent lung complications.

Procedure

1. Elevate the head of the bed 45 degrees, arms relaxed and, if necessary, pillow under knees; upper chest should remain relaxed.
2. Inhale slowly through the nose and let the "V" between the ribs rise.

3. Exhale slowly through the mouth (by pursing the lips) and relaxing the "V" between the ribs.

Lower Chest Breathing

Objective   This exercise, like diaphragm breathing, will maintain full, long expansion by expanding the lower lungs.

Procedure

1. Place your hand over lower ribs.
2. As you breathe in slowly, push the lower ribs against the firm pressure of your hands to fullest expansion.
3. At the end of the "breathe in," release the pressure of your hands and *hold the breath for a moment*. Then, breathe out slowly.
4. Can be repeated for upper chest by putting hand on either your shoulder or under your arm for Step 1 and repeating Steps 2 and 3.

Postural Drainage

Objective   By use of specific positions, allow the force of gravity to assist in the removal of bronchial secretions from the bronchioles into the bronchi and trachea by expectoration.

Procedure

1. If agents or medications are used, give prior to starting treatment.
2. Place patient so that diseased area(s) are in a near vertical position.
3. Positions assumed are determined by the location, severity, and duration of mucus obstruction. Upper lobes are usually drained by upright positions; lower and middle lobes are drained by head-down positions. (See Figure 4.1.)
4. Encourage diaphragmatic breathing throughout postural drainage exercises to help widen airways so secretions can be drained.
5. Encourage patient to cough after allotted time in each position.

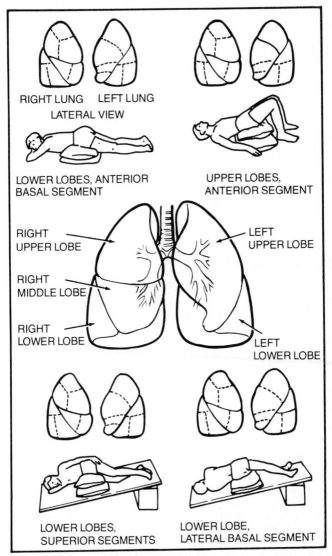

Figure 4-1: Postural Drainage Positions.

6. Chest wall percussion and vibration may be needed and should be ordered, if gravity positions are not fully successful.

   • Percussion—Movement done by striking chest wall in a rhythmical fashion with cupped hands over the area of the chest to be drained. The wrists are alternately flexed and extended so that the chest is cupped or clapped in a painless manner.
   • Vibration—Technique of applying manual compression and tremor to the chest wall during the exhalation phase of respiration.

7. Discontinue procedure if tachycardia, palpitations, dyspnea, chest pain, or other symptoms occur which may indicate hypoxemia.

8. Exercises are usually performed 2–4 times daily: before meals and at bedtime.

Bed Positions To Prevent Deformities— Long-Term Patient

Correct Back-Lying Position

• No pillow under head, entire head of bed may be raised if condition permits.
• Bed sheet covers outside end of bed, not tucked in.
• Foot board when any tendency to foot drop—4 in. space between end of mattress and board to prevent pressure buildup on heels.
• Firm support placed under back (folded towel or bath blanket) whenever a sag in the mattress is present will keep the back in a more normal position.
• Legs held in relaxed position without external rotation. Place sandbag/rolled blanket outside the leg mid-thigh to ankle.
• Small pillow or pad under knees *only* to prevent hyperextension.
• If arms are involved, support on pillow with *slight* shoulder abduction, elbow flexion, and hand supported by roll in position of function.

Correct Side-Lying Position

- Bed flat.
- Back or spine kept in straight line; avoid rotation.
- Pillow under head at proper height to prevent bend in neck.
- For the gap that is present between pelvic rim and ribs, place small pillow or blanket at area to provide minimal support, keeping spine straight.
- Full size pillow between legs to support top leg from upper thigh down.
- Never keep knees bent more than a right angle.
- Foot as close to right angle as possible, not left to dangle over end of pillow.
- Arms in comfortable position, forward from trunk with comfortable elbow bend. Top arm resting on rolled pillow will relieve pull on shoulder girdle and prevent rotation of trunk.
- Rolled pillows behind patient for support.

Correct Face-Lying Position

- Bed flat.
- No pillow under head.
- Toes over edge of mattress with soft padding under ankles. This will relieve pressure and produces a slight knee flexion, reducing strain in posterior knee region.
- One arm straight at side, other flexed, hand beside face, and face turned in direction of hand, or both arms may be bent.
- Bath blanket/small pillow under abdomen between ribs and pelvis to prevent hyperextension of spine.
- Small pads/folded towel under each shoulder to prevent forward shoulder rotation.

Correct Sitting Position

- Head of bed elevated with chin extended; be careful to keep head flexed.
- No pillows. If patient demands one, place under shoulders, not just head.

- Knees elevated by raising lower part of bed to position where patient will not slide down.
- Support feet properly to keep Achilles tendons (heel cords) stretched.
- Blanket/small pillow under small of back to prevent bowing of back. Avoid a thick blanket which leads to hyperextension.

Correct Position Changes

- The more time a bed patient can spend in a face lying position, the fewer deformities will occur.
- Gradually increase face lying position. The ultimate goal is four times per day for minimum of 1–2 hours if able to tolerate.
- Condition patient to sleep in face lying position.
- Should be in back lying position majority of time when not face lying.
- When turning patients on side for rest, position should not be maintained longer than one hour at any one time; 30 minutes is the optimum time. When patients are kept on side for longer than recommended, increased knee flexion, changes in hip flexion, and flattening of the lower back, all precursors for contractures, occur.
- When sitting patients on side of bed, be sure feet are supported on bedside chair, and patient sits with back straight, supported with pillows if necessary.

Moving the Dependent Patient in Bed

Rolling

- Bend knees and drop to side you are rolling to.
- Reach with opposite arm to side you are rolling to.

Movement to Head of Bed

- Bend knees, stabilize at ankles.
- Patient uses trapeze if available or reaches for head of bed.
- Simultaneously pull with arms while pushing feet against bed.

Lateral Movement

Lower Body   Knees bent, feet placed slightly off center to direction of movement. Patient lifts buttocks up and to the side.

Upper Body   Patient crosses arms, attempts partial sit up, and rocks to direction of desired movement.

Supine to Sit

- Use rolling method to come to side-lying position.
- Bend knees up and drop feet over side of bed and simultaneously push to sitting position.
- Place chair/commode at side of bed for patient to use for leverage, which will also decrease fear of falling.

Transfer Techniques

- Most transfers are made to the normal, stronger side regardless of the cause of disability.
- Begin teaching as soon as patient can balance in sitting position and assessment of lower extremity strength indicates sufficient strength to weight bear.
- If not enough strength to weight bear, consider using: sliding bar transfer, lift devices, wheelchair with removable arms and leg rests.

Sit to Stand

Used for walker, crutches, pivot transfer.

1. Slide to edge of seat.
2. Feet placed flat on the floor and under the body.
3. Push with the arms, leaning forward to raise the buttocks.
4. Stand erect.

Stand to Sit

1. Place seating area directly behind knees.
2. Reach one or both hands back to the object before bending knees to sit.
3. When steady, sit—avoid "plopping."

Pivot Transfer

1. Objects to sit upon placed at approximately 45° angle to each other.
2. Transfer *sit to stand* as before.
3. Reach to object headed to.
4. Twist buttocks to pivot and sit.

Range of Motion Exercises

Objectives   To prevent formation of adhesions, prevent shortening of muscle fibers and to preserve ROM.
   See Figures 4.2 through 4.7 for procedures.

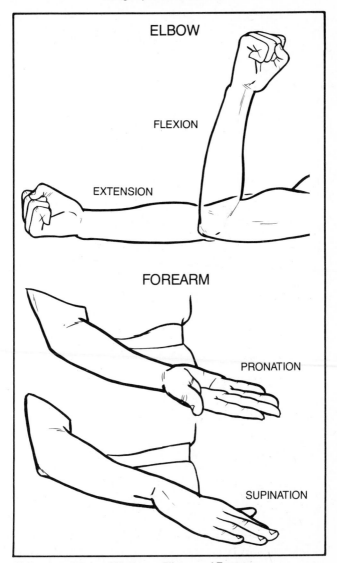

Figure 4-2: Range of Motion—Elbow and Forearm.

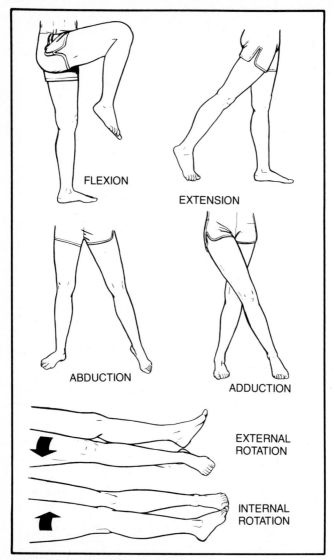

FLEXION

EXTENSION

ABDUCTION

ADDUCTION

EXTERNAL
ROTATION

INTERNAL
ROTATION

Figure 4-3: Range of Motion—Hip.

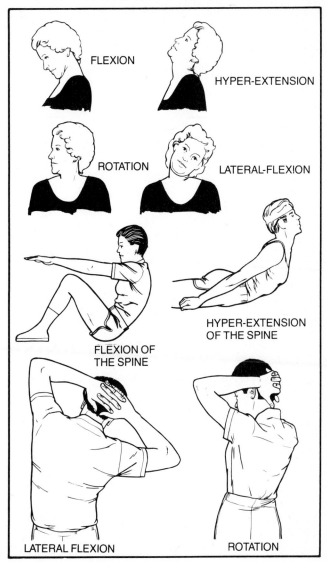

Figure 4-4: Range of Motion — Neck.

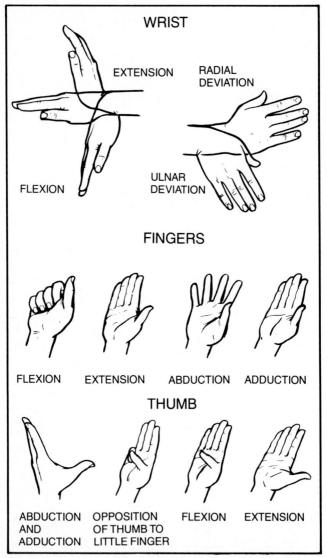

Figure 4-5: Range of Motion—Wrist, Fingers, Thumb.

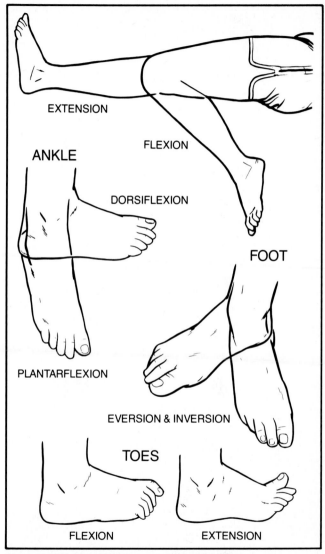

Figure 4-6: Range of Motion—Ankle, Foot, Toes.

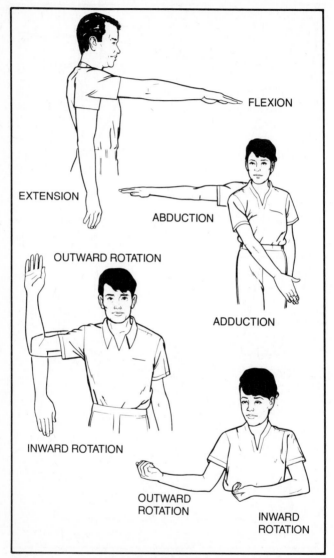

Figure 4-7: Range of Motion—Shoulder.

Ambulation with Assistive Devices

Preparatory Exercises for Ambulation with Assistive Devices

1. Bed and sitting exercises to include:

   - Full ROM for affected extremity.
   - Strengthening exercises for unaffected extremity.
   - Strengthening of muscles of shoulders, chest, arms, hands, back, and abdomen.
   - Balancing exercises.

2. Standing exercises as soon as possible to include:

   - Posture exercises.
   - Balancing exercises between two chairs.
   - Balancing exercises against wall.
   - Weight-shifting exercises.

Use of Crutches or Cane

MEASURING—CRUTCHES

1. Stand in good alignment with heels against wall. Extend tape measure from anterior fold of axilla to a point 6 inches out from the patient's heel.
2. If standing not possible use back-lying position in good alignment, arms straight at the side, feet should be at right angles, shoes on.
3. Hand bar should be placed so that elbows are slightly bent. Axillary bar padding is not necessary.
4. Wrists are to be held in hyperextension. (See Range of Motion—wrist extension.)
5. Weight is on the palms.
6. Crutch tips should be 1.5 in., suction type.
7. Shoes should be well fitting, low broad heels with good rubber lifts.

MEASURING—CANE

1. Measure from hip joint to 6 in. out from heel.
2. Use tip with suction cup.

WALKING

- Use one crutch or cane on the *unaffected side.*
- Crutch or cane is put forward at the same time with affected foot, thereby taking weight off that foot and equalizing balance.
- Stand tall with good posture and look ahead, not down at the feet.

UP STAIRS—"UP WITH THE GOOD"

1. Lead with the good foot.
2. Then, move the cane or crutch and the bad foot up the step at the same time.

DOWN STAIRS—"DOWN WITH THE WEAK"

1. Lead with the cane or crutch and the bad foot.
2. Bring the good foot down to the same step.
3. When using steps, use the railing with the free hand whenever possible.

THREE-POINT GAIT   may be taught:

1. When there is involvement of one extremity.
2. When order is for no weight bearing on one extremity.
3. When partial weight bearing is permitted.

Starting position is as shown in Figure 4.8.

SWING THROUGH GAIT   may be taught:

1. When three point gait has been mastered with ease.
2. When both lower extremities are paralyzed.
3. Pre-prosthetic amputee.

Starting position is as shown in Figure 4.9.

WALKER GAIT

1. Place walker forward so back legs of walker are even with patient's toes—remind patient not to put walker too far in front and, therefore, lose balance.
2. Progress one foot (the one which is weaker or painful) forward halfway into walker (see Figure 4.10).
3. Step so both feet are even. Body should not touch the front of walker.

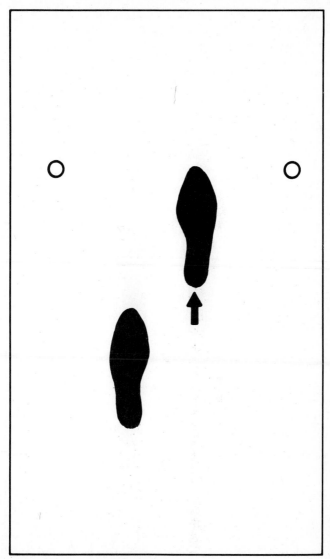

Figure 4-8: Three Point Gait.

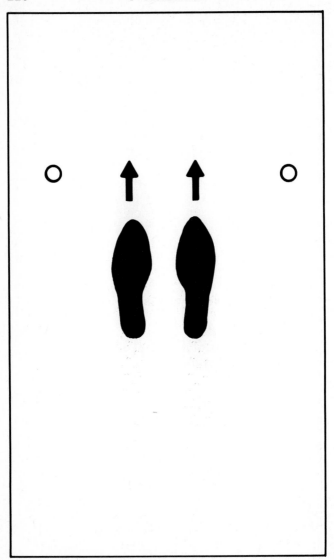

Figure 4-9: Swing Through Gait.

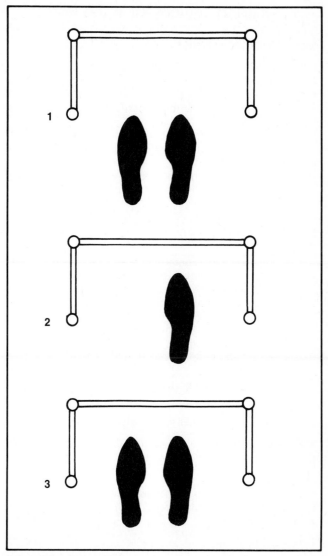

Figure 4-10: Walker Gait.

Sterilizing Equipment in the Home

Moist-Heat Sterilization

1. When boiling equipment, have a large pan with handles on both sides and a lid and use wide-mouth jars.
2. It is best to boil equipment about one hour before use. It then will be more sterile and cool enough to handle.
3. Always boil equipment covered with water in a covered pan. Start timing after water begins to boil and boil for 10 minutes.
4. If equipment won't be used for a while, keep the lid on the pan until ready for use.

Dry-Heat Sterilization

1. You can use any metal pan such as a cake or pie pan to sterilize dressings in the oven.
2. Place the clean dressings wrapped in a clean cloth into the pie tin and bake in a preheated oven at 350° for one hour. Wrap the cloth so that you will not contaminate the dressings upon unwrapping. Let cool slightly before using.

Solutions

Solutions Used as Disinfectants

Bleach—Undiluted   is used for spillage of body fluids, that is, blood, vomitus and excreta for patients with hepatitis.

Bleach—Diluted   in a mixture of 1:10 can be used for cleaning contaminated surfaces when caring for patients with AIDS.

Lysol Solution   should be mixed as directed on bottle. Never use anywhere near food; all items in contact with solution should be rinsed well.

White Vinegar in a mixture of 1:3 can be used to disinfect respiratory and tracheostomy equipment. First, wash equipment well with friction and soap and water. Place in vinegar solution and store in a closed container. Allowed to air dry before using.

Solutions for Wounds and Irrigations

Although solutions used for dressing changes and some irrigation procedures can be purchased already prepared and sterilized, often patient situations demand that these solutions be made in the home. High cost, lack of financial resources, long-term use, and lack of transportation to purchase supplies often mean that the nurse can best assure that procedures are complied with if she teaches families how to make their own solutions in the home.

In the following section, procedures for making and storing solutions in the home are given in a simple format that can be easily taught to patients. Once a procedure is established, solutions can be made in the home easily and without danger to the patient as well as saving a great deal of money. Things to remember when using solutions in the home are:

- Teach the family the difference between sterile and clean technique.
- Use a safe container such as canning jars, mayonnaise jars, and such.
- Label all solutions with name and date prepared.
- Keep solutions out of reach of small children and pets.

Sterile Water A new container of sterile water should be made daily, and the solution in the jar should be stored in a cool place.

EQUIPMENT Large pan with a lid, small-mouth glass jar with a lid (1 quart size, a mayonnaise jar is a good choice), tap water.

PROCEDURE

1. Fill the jar to the top with tap water.
2. Stand jar up in the pan and fill up the pan with enough water to cover the jar. Drop the jar lid into the pan and be sure it sinks to the bottom.
3. Cover the pan, bring the water to a boil, and boil for 20 minutes.
4. After the 20 minutes, remove from heat, cool and pour off enough water from the pan that you can handle the jar comfortably or use tongs that have also been boiled. Touching only the outside of the jar, take the jar out of the pan and set it on a counter.
5. Pour off the remaining water in the pan, remove the jar lid, touching only the outside of the rim and place it on the jar. Note: This procedure can be followed to prepare an empty sterile jar and lid. Water can be boiled in another container and poured into the sterile empty jar, the lid attached and water stored.

Normal Saline   Normal saline is simply water that has a certain amount of salt in it that is compatible with all body fluids. If you are using the normal saline for a bladder irrigation or other sterile procedure make a new supply every day. If it is used for a clean dresssing or other clean procedure, it will keep refrigerated for one week.

EQUIPMENT   Table salt—iodized or noniodized—tap water, teaspoon, measuring cup, quart jar with lid and pan.

STRENGTH   Normal Saline: 0.9%

PROCEDURE

1. Wash teaspoon, measuring cup, jar, and lid in hot soapy water and rinse well in hot water.
2. Boil at least six (6) cups of tap water in a pan for 20 minutes and let cool.
3. Pour four (4) cups of the boiled water into a clean jar.
4. Add two (2) teaspoons of salt and mix well with the water.

5. Put the lid on the jar, write the date you made the solution on the outside of the jar, and put in the refrigerator.

Dakin's Solution　Dakin's solution can be made from bleach. Bleach is 5.25% sodium hypochlorite and full strength Dakin's solution is 0.5% sodium hypochlorite. The solution is good only for seven (7) days since it deteriorates.

EQUIPMENT　Clorox, sterile water (*see* page 231), a pint glass jar with cover, and a teaspoon that has been sterilized.

STRENGTH　Half Strength (0.25) = 25 cc per pint of sterile water
Full Strength (0.50) = 50 cc per pint of sterile water

PROCEDURE

1. Into the sterile jar, put the amount of Clorox desired to achieve the strength ordered.
2. Add enough sterile water to fill to the top. The water does not have to be cooled before adding to the bleach if the solution is to be used immediately. If the solution is to be stored, it is preferable to cool the water before adding to the bleach.
3. Cover with a sterile lid and store in a cool place.

Chloramine T (Chlorazene)　This solution is similar to Dakin's Solution in terms of activity. It is more stable and lasts longer but should not be used in place of Dakin's Solution without the permission of the physician. It is used in 1% or 2% solutions applied in the same manner as Dakin's Solution. You must have Chlorazene tablets (purchased by prescription) to make this solution.

EQUIPMENT　Chlorazene tablets, sterile water, and a small container.

STRENGTH　1% Chlorazene-1 tablet to 1 oz. water
2% Chlorazene-2 tablets to 1 oz. water

Procedure   Mix together in small, clean container.

Acetic Acid   Acetic acid can be made with white vinegar since vinegar contains 5% acetic acid. Acetic acid may be used for dressings but should not be used for bladder irrigations since the acid can cause a negative effect on kidney functioning. Even though the solution can be kept in the refrigerator one week, a fresh solution made every day is best.

Equipment   White distilled vinegar, sterile water, 1.5 qt or glass bowl. Jar with cover, tablespoon, measuring cup, and large pan.

Strength   0.25 acetic acid = 4 tablespoons vinegar in 5 cups of boiled water.

Procedure

1. Wash tablespoon, measuring cup, jar, and lid in hot, soapy water. Rinse well in hot water.
2. Boil at least six (6) cups of water in the pan for 20 minutes and let it cool.
3. Add four (4) tablespoons of white, distilled vinegar, and mix well.
4. Put the lid on the jar and write the date you made it on a label on the outside of the jar.

5

Helpful Hints and Improvised Equipment

Nurses working in the home have long been the master of improvising techniques and equipment to effectively care for patients in less than optimal surroundings. A practical handbook for the home care nurse must include hints that can be shared among nurses and patients as care is delivered in the home.

The hints listed here have been gathered from patients, their families, and from the experiences of nurses. I hope that as more are developed they can be shared through subsequent editions of this handbook.

Helpful Hints

Support Groups

The use of Support Groups is one of the most helpful hints patients and families can be given. Self-help and family support groups can be found that provide a mechanism for people with certain diseases, limitations, or experiences to share problems, solutions, and support. Referring patients to these groups can help teach coping strategies for patients and families alike. Some states have developed directories of self- and mutual-help support groups available through community resources.

General Hints

- Inexpensive gowns can be made for patients by using an old, man-tailored shirt that has the cuffs and collar removed. A row of snaps or velcro can be sewn to the button placket for ease in removing. Also an old over-sized cotton T-shirt can also be used. Since these are cotton they are washed easily and are comfortable to the patient.

- Sticky tape such as masking tape or decals used for bottoms of bathtubs can be put on the bottom of bedroom slippers to keep a patient from slipping.
- A washcloth can be used to open a tightly screwed on jar lid.
- Meat tenderizer paste—0.5 tsp. of meat tenderizer to 2 tsp. water—is helpful to draw poison out of bee sting.
- Always try to use equipment a patient has in the home rather than purchasing expensive items. Ideas for alternative items include:

    1. Plastic trash bags as mattress protectors.
    2. Rolled towels in place of air rings.
    3. Rolled blankets under a mattress for elevation in place of an expensive foam wedge.
    4. A thick pile rug rather than an expensive bed fluff.

- Plastic or wooden golf tees can be used as a clamp for a feeding tube that must be clamped between feedings.
- Smoke Detectors can be used as a "call bell." The patient can press the test button and the noise can be heard from a long distance. This is especially helpful when patient needs to be heard from various floors of the home.

Laryngectomy Patients

Have someone tape record several "emergency" phone messages that could be played over the phone to the police, fire department, ambulance service, physician, or other contact people. Each tape should be separate and marked clearly for fast use and kept by the phone with a list of the corresponding emergency phone numbers. The message should include their name, address, phone number, the assistance needed, and the name and address of a friend or relative.

Ostomy Care

- When caring for a colostomy patient, it is easier while they are changing their bag and/or doing an irrigation for them to sit backward on the toilet seat. This allows them to have a more stable, comfortable position as well as they can use the back of the toilet as a flat area to place supplies.
- If an ileostomy patient experiences difficulty changing their pouch due to the constant runny stools, eating 6 marshmallows 30 minutes before removing the pouch can cut down on gastric motility, making the appliance change easier.
- Appliances with a pectin or karaya base should be kept in a cool, dark place since they melt in extreme heat. In warm weather, appliances don't wear as long as in cold weather. Use of an electric blanket can melt the appliance.
- Patients can keep on hand an "emergency kit" so they are prepared when their pouches or sites leak. This kit would include a pair of underwear, stoma bag, a small facecloth or premoistened towelettes, and a small, plastic bottle of deodorant. Men can use a shaving kit and women a makeup bag that can be inconspicuously placed in a car's glove compartment or anywhere else the patient might find convenient.
- To help the patient learn how to change the bag efficiently and inspect the stoma, use a mirror when changing the appliance. A wall mirror installed in the bathroom can be very helpful.
- A few drops of baby oil put into the opening in the bottom of the pouch will make it easier to empty the contents.
- *Do not use* aspirin in the pouch to control odors—this can cause bleeding of the stoma; likewise, *do not* punch holes in the pouch to relieve gas build up. Holes in the pouch destroy the odor barrier properties of the pouch. There are gas-odor filters widely available and mouthwash can be used to rinse the bag.
- To make stoma pads, buy a box of 12 disposable diapers (over 12-lb size), gently flatten out, and cut in

quarters, or halves if a large one is needed. Bind the
cut ends with Micropore tape so as not to leak cotton.
This small investment can yield 48 moistureproof pads
for a colostomy.

- Men who have problems with post-op discomfort while
  trying to wear belts are wise to wear suspenders that
  produce less pressure on the abdominal area.

- If irrigating and traveling out of the country or camping, water used for irrigation must be safe to drink.
  Halazone tablets may be purchased to purify the water.
  Irrigation times should remain the same when traveling.

- The United Ostomy Association should be shared as
  a valuable resource to all patients. Members receive
  the ostomy quarterly magazine to keep up to date on
  product information, local suppliers throughout the
  country, and a directory of enterostomal therapists.
  The address is: United Ostomy Association, Inc., 2001
  West Beverly Blvd., Los Angeles, CA 90057.

Cataract Patients

- Cataract patients are often instructed post-op to remain still for 4–6 weeks without straining, reading,
  or watching television. To provide activity during these
  quiet periods—because these periods can increase
  anxiety—encourage the family or patient preopera-
  tively to obtain "talking books." These can be either
  borrowed from the local library, the society for the
  prevention of blindness, or can now be purchased in
  major book and department stores. This, with a small
  tape recorder or record player, can help the patient be
  entertained while resting.

- If a cataract patient has more than one type of eyedrop
  to take, each bottle should have a different colored
  bottle and/or label with the time and the number of
  drops clearly marked. This makes it easier for the patient and family to distinguish the difference and follow through with directions.

Patients with Casts

- To keep casts clean on upper extremities, cut off the tube part of a white sock and place it over the cast. This can be washed and changed every day at minimal expense.
- A patient with a long leg cast can use a cloth elbow sling with an attached strap. The sling is placed around the affected foot and the straps attached by a pin or tape to the knee area which is easy to reach. The patient can then hold onto the strap, which supports the lower leg, and is able to lift the affected leg easily to maneuver in bed or in a wheelchair.

Bedbound Patients

- A rope can be attached to the end of the bed frame so that patients can be assisted in pulling themselves up while lying down. It is important that the rope be placed on the *opposite* side of the bed that the patient gets into so better leverage can occur.
- A pie plate can be used for a small bed pan for a child in a Spica cast.
- Knee rests can be improvised by rolling sheets, blanket sheets, or blankets and placing them below a patient's knee(s), in addition to a pillow placed under the knees.
- Heel and elbow protectors can be made from strips of absorbent cotton that has been twisted into the shape of a donut and closed with adhesive tape.
- Worn out socks can be used as elbow protectors. Cut off the leg portion, fold it in half, and slip on as an elbow guard. Cotton is the best choice since it is cooler and easier to wash.

Patients with Diarrhea

- Gelatin water can be used for diarrhea and vomiting to replace fluids and calories.

Diarrhea Diet (Adult)   Clear fluids for 12–24 hours (water, 7-Up or ginger ale, Gatorade, tea, or broth). If diarrhea has stopped, advance to selected solids, such as, nonsweetened cereals of rice or corn, bread, (not whole grain), macaroni, potatoes, rice, yellow vegetables (squash or carrots), light-colored fruits (apples or bananas), and meats. No dairy products for 3 to 6 days.

Diarrhea Diet (Pediatric) Clear fluids for 12–24 hours (Gatorade, 7-Up or ginger ale, water, weak tea); Pedialyte for infants. When diarrhea has stopped, advance to soy formula diluted with twice the amount of water called for on the can; increase concentration to full strength over a 24-hour period, then advance to select solids as listed in the adult diet. Withhold dairy products for 3–6 days. If the child is not on formula, advance to rice cereal, bananas, yellow vegetables, clear fluids as listed for beverage after 24 hours on clear liquids.

Enemas

- Always place a patient on their left side when giving an enema.
- Many patients, especially the elderly, often have difficulty retaining enemas due to lack of muscle control. A suggestion: Cut the tip off a baby bottle nipple and insert the enema tube through the nipple. When the tube is inserted in the patient, the nipple rim surrounds the anus and acts as a sphincter.

Sitz Bath

A patient should lie down for at least 30 minutes after a sitz bath. During the procedure, the very vascular area of the rectum becomes filled with blood. When the procedure is completed and the patient stands up they can get orthostatic hypotension from the lack of blood supply to their head. Lying down for 30 minutes will help relieve the lightheadedness and vertigo that can happen after a sitz bath.

Catheterizing

Often women, especially the elderly, find the traditional dorsal recumbant position for catheterization uncomfortable. A more comfortable position is: the patient on their left side in Sims position, with right knee and thigh drawn up, if possible. Place a sterile drape over the buttocks, covering the rectal area and then spread the labia and proceed with the catheterization.

Stroke Patients

- Cooking utensils and measuring spoons with flat bottoms are more stable for pouring ingredients. Perforated spoons or ladles make it easier for the person to lift food from hot liquid.
- Enlarging handles make eating utensils easier to hold. A sponge rubber hair roller (the kind with a hold through the middle) placed over the handle of common silverware is an example of this.
- Available devices that can be purchased in stores: an egg separator, opener for screw-on lids, a pizza cutter to cut food, a small cutting board that has an edge around it (similar to a picture frame) can be used to secure things like bread that needs to be buttered.
- A damp washcloth placed under a plate/dish can prevent slippage during one-handed cutting.
- For any patient who has limited mobility anything he or she needs should be placed at waist height.
- A patient who has hemiparesis (limited movement on one side) should always put their weak arm or leg into the garment first when getting dressed and then should undress by removing the strong arm or leg first.
- Patients with hemiparesis who also have vision problems may want to put makeup on the unaffected side first to use as a guide for the affected side.

Patients with Poor Vision

- Don't overlook the somewhat obvious solution to improving the vision of patients with failing eyesight. Often putting in larger light bulbs, moving lights, or putting in lighter window coverings can make a big difference in their ability to see major items in a room.
- Patients with poor eyesight may be better able to be oriented to a room by placing a piece of colored glass on a window sill or a lamp or a colored light bulb left burning in a particular location in a room.

Diabetic Patients

When diabetics have difficulty remembering to take their daily insulin, they can tape a month from a calendar to their refrigerator. Not only do they see this first thing in the morning to remember their insulin but they can mark off the day after they inject themselves so they will be assured they took the dose.

Wounds

- Remind patients they can use a hair dryer to dry skin thoroughly. This is especially important in obese patients and any where else that drying well with a towel might be difficult or painful. The heat setting should always be on low and keep the dryer always moving to facilitate air circulation.
- A small, 6-in. hem gauge that is marked in centimeters can be used to measure the size of wounds, or the area of drainage on a bandage. Carry one in your nursing bag.
- In females who need breast or sternal dressings, instead of using Montgomery straps, a binder, or tape, the patient's bra may be used. This holds the dressing in place, is more comfortable, and reduces skin irritation.
- When immobilizers or binders are used, especially those with Velcro bindings or fasteners, a disposable baby diaper liner can be used for padding to prevent skin irritation and breakdown. They are well padded and serve the purpose perfectly.
- Vaseline gauze can be made by using roller gauze and regular petroleum jelly. Accordian pleat (fold back and forth) the gauze in a metal mixing bowel or a shallow glass pan. Put a generous amount of petroleum jelly on top of the gauze, cover with aluminum foil and bake at 375° for 25 minutes. If sterile gauze is needed, individual aluminum foil packets can be made.

Medications

- When using medication that needs accurate measurement and patient is unable to see lines accurately on vial (such as working with medication in a nebulizer), use a medicine dropper, and have patient count by drops which is much easier.

- With time-released medications, advise patients not to open capsules and mix with food. This can change how the medication is absorbed and alter the dosage.
- When giving an injection in the hip, have the patient point his toes together. This will make it impossible for him to tense up his buttocks muscles,and the injection will be less painful.
- Daily doses of medications may be laid out for a patient with the aid of an egg carton. The cups may be labeled with the times the medications are to be taken and then the proper pills put in each cup. This is especially helpful for elderly patients living alone and can be taught to family members so they do not need to measure medications daily for the patient.
- For the most part, prescription drugs come labeled regarding how and when to be taken as well as foods or other substances to avoid. The following list will assist in guiding your patients when taking certain groups of drugs:

Drugs and Alcohol Alcohol should not be combined with hypotics, barbiturates, sedatives, CNS depressants, antihistamines and tranquilizers. It is usually a good idea to avoid alcohol consumption while taking drugs in general.

Drugs and Water Fluids should be forced when taking sulfa drugs such as Bactrim, Septra, Zyloprim (allopurinol), Metamucil, and ASA.

Anticoagulants ASA should never be taken with anticoagulants. Pharmacists should check to see of interactions of all drugs with anticoagulants.

Mineral Oil and Vitamins The elderly especially rely on assistance to keep regular bowel habits. They are also the population that takes the most vitamins per capita. If a patient takes mineral oil with vitamins it can diminish the effect of the vitamin.

Antacids   They can destroy the enteric coating on medications.

MAO Inhibitors   Mixing of these drugs with the following foods and medications can result in exceedingly elevated blood pressure causing stroke or death.

- **Foods** that interact negatively include foods high in tyramine such as: aged cheese, pickled herring, soy sauce, avocados, wild game, bananas, canned figs, chianti wine, chocolate, chicken livers, licorice, pineapple, raisins, raw yeast, sour cream, yogurt, meat extracts, and tenderizers.
- **Drugs** that interact negatively with MAO inhibitors include: Lomotil, Bovril, Marmite, nasal and pulmonary decongestants, sleeping or antiappetite medications, and antidepressants.
- **Diuretics and Steroids** Since they cause potassium depletion, supplements should be added to the diet in the form of medication and foods high in potassium (*See* list in Appendix D).
- **Drugs and the Sun.** An increased sensitivity to sunlight is caused by certain medications. Tetracycline is the most common.

Common Home Preparations

The following are common preparations used for a variety of problems. If appropriate, contact the physician or primary care provider before recommending a preparation to the patient.

Honey-Lemon Cough Mix

2 parts honey to 1 part lemon juice. 1 part alcohol (brandy, rum, vodka, and so on) may be added if desired. The honey soothes the throat and acts as an expectorant; lemon juice helps reduce the viscosity of phlegm; and the alcohol is an antitussive. This can be taken by the teaspoon p.r.n. for coughs for adults and older children. Younger children can use 1/4 tsp. Use light corn syrup instead of honey for children under 1 because botulism spores in honey may

cause problems with infants but do not affect older children.

Oatmeal Bath

Fill a thin cloth or the toe of an old nylon stocking with uncooked oatmeal flakes (about 1 cup), tie closed, and allow to float in a bathtub of tepid water. Or, cook the bag of oatmeal for 30 minutes then squeeze the bag in warm bath water to extract the gelatinous starch. A bath in this solution is often useful to reduce vaginal itching and skin irritations.

Saline Gargle or Mouthwash

¼ tsp. salt to 1 cup warm water.

Tea Bag Teether

Brew a cup of tea. After steeping, wring out the tea bag and let it cool. Let the infant chew on the moist bag. The tannic acid in the tea helps reduce inflammation in gums.

Vinegar Douche

1 Tbsp. white vinegar to 1 qt. tepid water. Thought to be helpful for yeast infections and other causes of vaginal itching although effectiveness is not proven.

Baking Soda Bath

Add a generous amount of baking soda (½ cup or more) to ½ tub of warm water.

Benadryl Maalox Mix

A solution of equal parts of Benadryl Elixir and Maalox to be used as a mouthwash or gargle for the relief of pain of oral herpes infections.

Cornstarch Bath

One handful of cornstarch added to a tub of tepid water or add ½ to 1 lb cornstarch to a pot of hot water, then add to bath; soak about 15 minutes. Useful to relieve itching and irritation.

Nutrition—Diet

Difficulty Swallowing   For patients past stroke or throat surgery, taking liquids is a problem. Freezing liquids, milk shakes, nutritional supplements, and eggnog can be helpful. Many liquids, even when unpleasant such as medication, are more easily tolerated when they are semi-solid.

Limited Fluid Restriction   Small quantities of liquid can be more satisfying to patients with fluid restrictions if they are frozen into "popsicles" from juice or an allowed supplement. If intake and output is important, measure the liquid into waxed paper cups with a stick in each and put in freezer. The cup can be removed by either running water over the outside or tearing off the paper cup. Foil cups or small plastic containers can also be used.

- If a patient uses a dietary supplement, instant breakfast mixes can often substitute for the more expensive prepared ones when prepared with whole milk. Check the labels on both to be sure the nutritional contents are similar (See list of supplements in Appendix J).
- Gatorade is a flavored drink good for replacing body fluids and chemicals lost through perspiration, diarrhea, or vomiting. Stokely Van Camp, bottlers of Gatorade, says that it is "essentially a 5% glucose solution that has 4.85 calories per ounce with the following electrolyte levels: sodium 21.0, potassium 2.5, chloride 17.0 and phosphate 6.8 milliequivalents per liter. A good idea is to freeze Gatorade into a popsicle. This is especially good for the elderly who have potential for electrolyte imbalance with nausea, vomiting or diarrhea.
- If a patient needs electrolytes orally and Gatorade is not available, or too costly, the following solution can be used after consulting with the physician. It is not especially tasty but can assist the patient in regaining an electrolyte balance.

1 tsp. salt
1 tsp. baking soda

3 cups strong black tea
1 cup water
Mix together all ingredients and chill.

Improvised Equipment

Bed Cradle

To alleviate the pressure of the covers over the feet of a bedbound patient try:

1. Laying a lightweight walker on the bed to support the covers.
2. Putting a small, open-legged television table under the covers with the tabletop facing the foot of the bed which can also be used as a footboard.
3. Using an empty cardboard box with the top cut off to allow the patient room to move feet.

Bed Table

- A bed table can be improvised by placing the longer end of an adjustable height ironing board across the bed.
- A bed table tray can be improvised with a cardboard or wooden box that has had the two wide sides cut out and then placed over the patients lap.

Footboards

When footboards are unavailable, high-topped canvas basketball sneakers work well at keeping the patient's feet aligned to prevent footdrop. They should be worn with cotton socks and rotated with a schedule of on 4 hours, off 4 hours to keep feet dry and healthy.

Bed Rails

A card table can be used as a bed rail for patients. Simply open two legs and slip them under the mattress. Make a soft cushion against the cardtable with pillows or blankets. This should not be used with a patient who is very active but can be extremely helpful when used to assure safety of the elderly or sedated patient.

Ice Collar

A wet dish towel frozen around a large cylinder (that is, a can) makes an effective ice collar. Wrap a cloth around a frozen juice can or put a frozen juice can in a sock and roll the can over a muscle in spasm.

Leg or Arm Life Exerciser

To make an inexpensive leg-lift or arm-lift exerciser, sew together the waistband of a man's cotton brief. Then slip the amount of weight ordered (can be 5 lb of sugar, plastic bag filled with rice or flour, and so on) into the brief through one leg hole. The patient puts the extremity to be exercised through one leg hole and out the other and moves the extremity up and down in the manner desired.

Appendices

A

1983 Metropolitan Height and Weight Tables

Men[1]

Height		Small Frame (lb)	Medium Frame (lb)	Large Frame (lb)
Ft	In			
5	2	128–134	131–141	138–150
5	3	130–136	133–143	140–153
5	4	132–138	135–145	142–156
5	5	134–140	137–148	144–160
5	6	136–142	139–151	146–164
5	7	138–145	142–154	149–168
5	8	140–148	145–157	152–172
5	9	142–151	148–160	155–176
5	10	144–154	151–163	158–180
5	11	146–157	154–166	161–184
6	0	149–160	157–170	164–188
6	1	152–164	160–174	168–192
6	2	155–168	164–178	172–197
6	3	158–172	167–182	176–202
6	4	162–176	171–187	181–207

[1]Weights are for ages 25–59 based on lowest mortality. Weight in pounds according to frame (in indoor clothing weighing approximately 5 lbs., shoes with 1-in. heels).

Women[2]

Height		Small Frame (lb)	Medium Frame (lb)	Large Frame (lb)
Ft	**In**			
4	10	102–111	109–121	118–131
4	11	103–113	111–123	120–134
5	0	104–115	113–126	122–137
5	1	106–118	115–129	125–140
5	2	108–121	118–132	128–143
5	3	111–124	121–135	131 –147
5	4	114–127	124–138	134–151
5	5	117–130	127–141	137–155
5	6	120–133	130–144	140–159
5	7	123–136	133–147	143–163
5	8	126–139	136–150	146–167
5	9	129–142	139–153	149–170
5	10	132–145	142–156	152–173
5	11	135–148	145–159	155–176
6	0	138–151	148–162	158–179

[2]Weights are for ages 25–59 based on lowest mortality. Weight in pounds according to frame (in indoor clothing weighing approximately 3 lbs., shoes with 1-in. heels).

Source of basic data for both tables: 1979 Build Study, Society of Actuaries and Association of Life Insurance Medical Directors of America, 1980.

B

Descriptors of Skin Lesions

1. Describe *where* on the body the lesion(s) is located:

   Face
   Face and shoulders and upper trunk
   Sun-exposed areas
   Dorsum of hands and forearms
   Linear following one nerve root
   Where clothing binds
   Moist folds where skin is against skin

2. Describe *how* the lesions are arranged:

   Annular = forming a ring
   Archiform = arcs
   Polycyclic = a combination of above
   Iris = looks like a bullseye
   Zosteriform = broad bands often following nerve
   Linear = streak

3. Describe the individual lesions.

Types of Primary Lesions

a. Diffuse color change such as erythema, gray-blue, brownish, yellow or depigmented.

b. Circumscribed, flat:
   macule = + 1 cm change in color, nonpalpable. Example: freckle.

c. Elevated, solid:

   Papule = <0.5 cm. Example: nevus
   Nodule = 0.5–2 cm
   Tumor = >2 cm

    Plaque = flat, elevated surface > 0.5 cm
    Wheal = irregular, transient skin edema

d. Superficial fluid filled:

    Vesicle = <0.5 cm, filled with serous fluid
    Bulla = >0.5 cm, filled with serous fluid
    Pustule = filled with pus
    Cyst = may appear as a nodule but opening reveals
        a deep, fluid filled cavity
    Vegetation = elevated, irregular growth
    Hyperkeratosis = keratotic elevations

Types of Secondary Lesions

Scale = thin plates of epithelium
Lichenification = dry area of hyperplasia with deep furrows
Crust = dried pus, blood, or serum
Atrophy = skin thin, smooth, and inelastic
Erosion = loss of superficial skin - surface is moist but doesn't bleed
Ulcer = depressed lesion, may bleed and scar
Fissure = cleavage or linear crack in skin

Common Lab Values

Blood Chemistry

Blood Urea Nitrogen (BUN)

Male: 10–25 mg/100 mL
Female: 8–20 mg/100 mL
Child: 8–18 mg/100 mL

Cholesterol

Adult: 120–260 mg/100 mL
Child: 5–100 mg/100 mL

Complete Blood Count

RBC:
Adult: 4–6 million cu mm (male)
4.2–5.4 million cu mm (female)
Child: Same after 2 years of age

RBC Indices:
MCV: 82–98 cu micron
MCHC: 32–36% or gm/100 mL
MCH: 27–31 pg

HCT:
Adult: 40–54% (male)
38–47% (female)
Child: 31–43%
Infant: 30–40%

HGB:
Adult: 13.5–18 gm/100 mL (male)
12–16 gm/100 mL (female)

Child: 11.2–13.4 gm/100 mL
Infant: 10–15 gm/100 mL

Platelets:
Adult: 150–400 thousand cu mm
Child: Same

WBC:
Adult: 4–11 thousand cu mm
Child: Same after 2 years of age

DIFF WBC:
(Adult and Child)
Neutrophils: 3–7 thousand or 54–62%
Eosinophils: 50–400 or 1–3%
Basophils: 25–100 or 0–1%
Lymphocytes: 1–4 thousand or 25–33%
Monocytes: 100–600 or 0–9%

Differential White Blood Count (Diff)

Neutrophils:
    Older Adult: 43–79%
    Adult: 32–62%
    Child: 30%
Band/Stabs: 3%
Eosinophils:
    Older Adults: 0–0.3%
    Adult: 1–3%
    Child: 2–3%
Basophils:
    Older Adult: 0–0.3%
    Adult: 6%
Lymphocytes:
    Older Adult: 11–48%
    Adult 25–33%
    Child: 30%
Monocytes:
    Older Adult: 1–15%
    Adult: 0–9%
    Child 5–8%

Digoxin/Digitoxin Toxicology Level

Digoxin (Therapeutic):
Adult: Below 2 ng/mL Child: Same
Digitoxin (Therapeutic): Below 30 ng/mL

Dilantin Toxicology/Level

Therapeutic level: 5–20 mcg/mL

Erythrocyte Count (RBC, Red Blood Count)

RBC:
Older Adult: 3–5 million/cu mm
Adult Female: 4–5.3 million/cu mm
Adult Male: 4.4–4.7 million/cu mm
Child: 4.6–4.8 million/cu mm

Fasting Blood Sugar or Glucose

Adult: 70–110 mg/100 mL
Child: 60–105 mg/100 mL

Glucose Tolerance (GTT)

FBS:
70–120 mg/100 mL in 30 minutes
155 mg/100 mL in 1 hour
165–180 mg/100 mL in 2 hours
14 mg/100 mL in 3 hours
80–120 mg/100 mL in 4 hours

Urine:
Negative for all urines

Hematocrit (Hct, Packed Red Cell Volume; PCV)

Adult: 40–54/100 mL (male)
      37–47/100 mL (female)
Child: 31–43/100 mL
Microhematocrit(Finger stick)
Adult: 45–47/100 mL (male)
      42–44/100 mL (female)
Child: 35–39/100 mL

Partial Thromboplastin Time (PTT, Activate PTT, APTT)

PTT: 30–45 seconds
APTT: 16–25 seconds

Prothrombin Time (PT, Pro-Time)

11–15 seconds or 100%; Each lab will differ

Sodium (Na$^+$)

137–142 mEq/L

Triglycerides (Lipids)

Adult: 20–150 mg/100 mL
Geriatric: 20–200 mg/100 mL

Uric Acid

Male: 2.1–7.8 mg/dL
Female: 2.0–6.4 mg/dL

Hemoglobin (HGB)

Older Adult: 10–17 gm/100 mL
Adult: 12–15 gm/100 mL (female)
      13–17 gm/100 mL (male)
Child: 12.5–13 gm/100 mL
Infant: 11.2–14 gm/100 mL
Hgb S: Negative

Urinalysis

Specific Gravity 1.010–1.022
Color: Clear
Glucose: Negative
Ketones: Negative
Blood: Negative
Protein: Negative
Bile: Negative
Bilirubin: Negative

Casts: Occasional hyaline
RBC: Negative
Crystals: Negative
WBC: Negative
pH: 5.0—8.0

Urine Culture

Negative or <10,000 organisms/mL

Urine Glucose

Random Urine: 0–15 mg/100 mL
24 hour urine: 100 mg/100 mL

Miscellaneous

Wound Culture
Normal Flora: Candida allbicans, Escherichia coli, Mycobacterium, Staphylococcus, Streptococcus.

Pulmonary Function Tests

Total Lung Capacity: 5500 mL
Vital Capacity: 4000–4800 mL
Residual Volume: 1200–1500 mL
Expiratory Reserve: 1200–1500 mL
Forced Vital Capacity: 4800 mL
Inspiratory Capacity: 2500–3600 mL

Note: There may be a slight variation in test results between laboratories. If any questions arise check the specific lab for their normal ranges.

Adapted from: Jaffe, M. and L. Skidmore *Diagnostic And Laboratory Cards for Clinical Use.* Bowie, Md.: Robert J. Brady, Company, 1984. Used with Permission.

Foods High in Potassium: Acceptable for Low-Sodium Diets

The following foods provide approximately 200 mg or 5 milliequivalents of potassium in the amount listed.

Food	Serving	Calories
Fruits		
Apricots,		
canned in juice	3 med. halves	40
dried	6 lg. halves	60
nectar	3/4 cup	120
Avocado	1/8 pear	45
Banana	4 inch piece	50
Dates	5	90
Fruit Cocktail	1/2 cup	45
Grapefruit Juice	1/2 cup	40
Nectarine	1/2 medium	20
Melon		
Cantaloupe	1/6 of 5 in. melon	30
Honeydew	1/6 of 5 in. melon	50
Orange	1 small	40
Peach	1 medium	40
Pear	1 medium	40
Prunes, cooked	5 medium	90
Prune Juice	1/3 cup	60
Raisins	3 Tablespoons	60
Strawberries, fresh	1 cup	55
Watermelon	1 1/4 cup	50

Food	Serving	Calories
Vegetables		
Asparagus	8 spears, 3/4 cup	35
Beans, cooked:		
Kidney, lima, white	1/3 cup	65
Green, snap	1 cup	35
Beet Greens, cooked	1/2 cup	25
Broccoli		
raw	1/2 sm. stalk	10
cooked	1/2 cup	25
Brussel Sprouts, cooked	1/2 cup	25
Cabbage, raw shredded	1 cup	20
Carrots		
raw	1 small	20
cooked	2/3 cup	45
Cauliflower (raw or cooked)	3/4 cup	20
Celery, raw	1/2 cup	25
Chickpeas (Garbanzos)	1/3 cup	120
Collards, cooked	1/2 cup	25
Cucumber	5 inch	25
Eggplant, cooked	1/2 cup	25
Lentils, cooked	1/2 cup	70
Mushrooms, raw	2/3 cup	15
Mustard greens, cooked	2/3 cup	20
Parsnips, cooked	1/3 cup	30
Potatoes, white		
baked	1/4 medium	20
boiled	1 small	70
Spinach		
cooked	1/3 cup	30
raw	3/4 cup	20
Split peas, cooked	1/2 cup	70
Squash, winter, baked	1/3 cup	50
Sweet potato, baked	1/2 medium	70
Tomato		
raw	1 medium	20
cooked	1/3 cup	15
Turnips (rutabaga)	2/3 cup	20

Other foods—It is important to continue including these protein foods which are also good potassium sources.

Protein Foods		
Beef, Medium fat	2 ounces	146
Chicken	2 ounces	146

Food	Serving	Calories
Fish, fresh,		
flounder, halibut		
perch, sole,		
pollock	2 ounces	110
Peanut butter, unsalted	2 Tablespoons	190
Peanuts, unsalted Virginia	20 nuts	90
Spanish	40 nuts	90
Pork, medium fat	2 ounces	146
Shellfish		
clams	5 large	55
scallops	5 large	55

References: Agriculture Handbook, No. 456

E

Low-Saturated Fat/Low-Cholesterol Diets

Foods Allowed	Foods to Avoid
Eggs—Three egg yolks/week	Eggs—Baked products high in egg yolks
Cholesterol-free egg subsitute	More than three egg yolks per week
Bread—White or whole grain bread English muffins Graham crackers/saltines Homemade breads with oils	Commercial biscuits Waffles and sweet rolls Flavored crackers Commercial mixes with dried egg
Milk—Fortified skim milk Non-fat dry milk 1% milk Low-fat yogurt Skim-milk buttermilk	Whole milk and 2% milk Evaporated whole milk Buttermilk Cream (Half and Half/sour cream) Whipping cream Nondairy coffee creamers Cheeses
Meat—Poultry, fish, and veal Shellfish Skim-milk cheese Oil-fried veal and fish Dried beans and peas Nonhydrogenated peanut butter	Fried meats Heavily marbeled meats Cold cuts/salt pork/bacon Canned meats Pork and beans Peanut butter Macadamia nuts

Foods Allowed	Foods to Avoid
Potatoes—White or sweet Rice or grits	Potato chips Egg noodles
Popcorn made with oil	Commercial popcorn
Macaroni-Spa- ghetti	

Soups—Fat-free broth and
          boullion
        Homemade Cream
          soup with skim
          milk
	Canned broth
	Soups made with whole milk
	Commercial cream soups

Desserts—Fruits
          Homemade pud-
            ding made with
            skim milk
	Commercial cakes, pies
	Cookies
	Doughnuts
	Ice Cream
	Coconut
	Canned pudding

Quick Diabetic Exchange Guide

	Calories		
	1200	1500	1800
Protein, 20% Calories	65	76	89
Fat, 30% Calories	39	50	64
Carbohydrate, 50% Calories	145	189	220
Total Calories	1207	1510	1812

Exchanges	B	L	S	HS	Total
1200 Calorie Diet					
Milk, 1% fat	1			1	2
Bread	1	2	1	1	5
Fruit	1	1	2		4
Vegetable		1	1		2
Meat		2 lean	3 med		5
Fat	1	2	1		4
1500 Calorie Diet					
Milk, 1% Fat	1			1	2
Bread	2	2	2	1	7
Fruit	2	1	1	1	5
Vegetable		1	1		2
Meat		2 lean	3 med	1 med	6
Fat	1	2	1		4
1800 Calorie Diet					
Milk, 1% fat	1	1/2	1/2	1/2	2 1/2
Bread	2	2	2	2	8
Fruit	1	2	2	1	6
Vegetable		1	1		2
Meat	1	2 lean	3 med	1 lean	7
Fat	1	2	2	1	6

Key: B = breakfast   L = lunch   S = supper   HS = bedtime

G

Food Sources of Major Vitamins

Food	Portion Size	Amount of Vitamin
		IU/Portion
Vitamin A—Adult RDA = 5000 IU		
Meats		
Beef Liver, fried	3.5 oz	50,375
Calf liver, cooked	3.5 oz	26,782
Chicken liver, cooked	2 Livers	25,760
Vegetables		
Potatoes, sweet, baked	1 medium	14,600
Carrots, raw	1 large	11,000
Spinach, raw	3.5 oz	8,100
Carrots, cooked	1/2 cup	8,000
Spinach, cooked	1/2 cup	7,300
Pumpkin, cooked	1/2 cup	8,000
Mustard greens, cooked	1/2 cup	5,800
Collard greens, cooked	1/2 cup	5,400
Turnip greens, cooked	1/2 cup	4,800
Squash, winter	1/2 squash	4,200
Broccoli, cooked	1/2 cup	1,900
Lettuce, romaine	4 leaves	1,900
Lettuce, iceberg	1/4 head	970
Asparagus, cooked	5–6 medium	900
Tomatoes, raw	1 small	900
Fruits		
Watermelon	1/16 melon (10 × 16 in.)	5,310
Cantaloupe	1/4 melon	3,400

Apricots, dried	4 halves	2,275
Apricots, raw	2–3 medium	2,700
Papaya, raw	1/3 medium	1,750
Nectarines, raw	1 medium	1,650

Riboflavin—Adult RDA = 1.2–1.7 mg		**mg/Portion**
Meats		
Beef liver, fried	3.5 oz	3.46
Calf liver, cooked	3.5 oz	3.34
Chicken liver, cooked	2 livers	1.77
Veal roast, cooked	3.5 oz	0.25
Beef, ground, cooked	3.5 oz	0.21
Egg, boiled	1 medium	0.13
Cereal products		
Barley cereals	1/2 cup	0.49
Dairy Products		
Milk, whole	1 cup	0.42
Cheese		
Cottage, creamed	1/3 cup	0.25
Blue or Roquefort	1 oz	0.17
Brick	1 oz	0.13
Cheddar	1 oz	0.13
Ice Cream	1/2 cup (1 scoop)	0.14
Vegetables		
Collard Greens, cooked	1/2 cup	0.20
Spinach, raw	3 1/2 oz	0.20

(Continued)

Appendix G—Continued

Food	Portion Size	Amount of Vitamin
Broccoli, cooked	1/2 cup	0.15
Asparagus, cooked	5–6 medium	0.18
Brussels sprouts, cooked	1/2 cup	0.11
Mustard greens, cooked	1/2 cup	0.14
Spinach, cooked	1/2 cup	0.13
Miscellaneous		
Brewer's yeast	1 Tbsp	0.34
Thiamin—Adult RDA = 1.0–1.5 mg		**mg/Portion**
Meats		
Pork Chops, cooked	3.5 oz	0.96
Ham, fresh, cooked	3.5 oz	0.58
Beef liver, fried	3.5 oz	0.24
Nuts		
Brazil	1/4 cup	0.82
Pecans	1/4 cup	0.18
Cashews	1/4 cup	0.11
Cereal products		
Barley cereals	1/2 cup	0.65
Wheat Germ	1 tbsp	0.20
Oatmeal, cooked	1/2 cup	0.11
Vegetables		
Green peas, cooked	1/2 cup	0.21

Soybeans, cooked	1/2 cup	0.21
Asparagus, cooked	5–6 medium	0.16
Beans, cooked		
Lima	1/2 cup	0.14
White	1/2 cup	0.14
Kidney	1/2 cup	0.14
Corn on cob, cooked	4-in. ear	0.12
Miscellaneous		
Brewer's yeast	1 Tbsp	1.25

Vitamin C—Adult RDA = 60 mg

		mg/Portion
Vegetables		
Green pepper, raw	1 large	128
Broccoli, cooked	1/2 cup	68
Brussels sprouts, cooked	1/2 cup	66
Spinach, raw	3.5 oz	51
Mustard greens, cooked	1/2 cup	48
Cabbage, raw	1 cup	47
Collard greens, cooked	1/2 cup	46
Parsley, raw	2 tbsp	34
Spinach, cooked	1/2 cup	25
Tomatoes	1 small	23
Potatoes, white, baked	1 small	20
Fruits		
Acerola	3.5 oz	1300
Oranges	1 medium	80

(Continued)

Appendix G—Continued

Food	Portion Size	Amount of Vitamin
Strawberries	10 large	59
Papayas, raw	1/3 medium	56
Lemons, peeled	1 medium	53
Grapefruit	1/2 medium	38
Limes, peeled	1 medium	37
Kumquats, raw	5–6 medium	36
Cantaloupe	1/4 medium	33
Tangerines	1 large	31
Honeydew melon	1/4 small	23

Niacin—Adult RDA = 13–19 mg

		mg/Portion
Meats		
Calf liver, cooked	3.5 oz	15.8
Beef liver, fried	3.5 oz	13.7
Chicken liver, cooked	2 livers	9.4
Chicken, cooked	3.5 oz	8.8
Beef, ground, cooked	3.5 oz	5.4
Haddock, cooked	3.5 oz	3.2
Nuts		
Peanuts, roasted	3 Tbsp	7.5
Peanut butter	2 Tbsp	4.8
Vegetables		
Green peas, cooked	1/2 cup	1.7

Potatoes, white, baked	1 small	1.7
Asparagus, cooked	5–6 medium	1.4
Corn on cob, cooked	4-in. ear	1.4
Black-eyed peas	3.5 oz	1.4
Lima beans, cooked	1/2 cup	1.0
Collard greens, cooked	1/2 cup	1.2
Miscellaneous		
Brewer's Yeast	1 Tbsp	3.0

Folic Acid—Adult RDA = 400 µg

		µg/Portion
Meats		
Beef liver	3.5 oz	290
Chicken liver	2 livers	230
Vegetables		
Asparagus	5–6 medium	89–140
Turnip greens	1/2 cup	63
Spinach	1/2 cup	49–110
Kale	1/2 cup	34
Endive	20 long leaves	27–63
Broccoli	1/2 cup	26
Escarole	4 large leaves	26

Vitamin B6—Adults RDA = 2.0–2.2 mg

		mg/Portion
Meats		
Beef liver	3.5 oz	0.8
Pork	3.5 oz	0.5
		(Continued)

Appendix G—Continued

Food	Portion Size	Amount of Vitamin
Beef round	3.5 oz	0.4
Chicken		
light	3.5 oz	0.7
dark		
Halibut	3.5 oz	0.4
Tuna	3.5 oz	0.4
Vegetables		
Beans, dry		
soy	1/2 cup	0.8
navy	1/2 cup	0.6
lentils	1/2 cup	0.6
garbanzo	1/2 cup	0.5
black eyed peas	1/2 cup	0.5
Potatoes	1 cup, diced	0.4
Spinach, raw	4 oz	0.3
Kale, raw	4 oz	0.3
Tomato juice	1 cup	0.5
Broccoli, raw	3 stalks	0.9
Asparagus, raw	12–14 spears	0.3
Corn, canned, cooked	1 cup	0.4
Cereals		
Rice Bran	1/4 cup	0.8
Wheat germ	1/4 cup	0.3

Brewer's yeast	1 tbsp	0.2
Whole wheat bread	1 slice	0.04
Dairy products		
Milk, whole	1 cup	0.1
Cottage Cheese	1 cup	0.1
Fruits		
Avocado	1/2 medium	0.45
Banana	1 medium	0.61
Raisins	1 cup	0.35
Nuts		
Walnuts	4–7 halves	0.1

Vitamin B12—Adult RDA = 3.0 µg

		µg/Portion
Meats		
Beef liver	3.5 oz	31–120
Beef round	3.5 oz	3.4–4.5
Ham	3.5 oz	0.9–1.6
Haddock	3.5 oz	0.6
Egg, whole	1 egg	0.7–1.2
Dairy products		
Milk, whole	1 cup	0.3
Cheese		
Swiss	1 oz	0.3
American	1 oz	0.2

SOURCE: Krause, Marie V. and Kathleen L. Mahan Food, Nutrition and Diet Therapy: A Textbook of Nutritional Care, 7th Edition. W.B. Saunders Co., 1984. Used with Permission.

Food Sources of Major Minerals

Food	Portion Size	Amount of Mineral
		mg/Portion
Calcium— Adults RDA = 800 mg		
Dairy Products		
Milk, whole	1 cup	288
Cheese		
Swiss	1 oz	248
Cheddar	1 oz	211
Brick	1 oz	204
Cottage, creamed	1/3 cup	94
Blue or Roquefort	1 oz	88
Ice Cream	1/2 cup (1 scoop)	84
Vegetables		
Collard greens, cooked	1/2 cup	152
Turnip greens, cooked	1/2 cup	140
Mustard greens, cooked	1/2 cup	138
Spinach, cooked	1/2 cup	83
Broccoli, cooked	1/2 cup	67
White beans, cooked	1/2 cup	50
Cabbage, raw	1 cup	49
Kidney beans, cooked	1/2 cup	48
Lima Beans, cooked	1/2 cup	38
Carrots, raw	1 large	37
Fruits		
Prunes	8 large	90
		(Continued)

Appendix H—Continued

Food	Portion Size	Amount of Mineral
		mg/Portion
Oranges	1 medium	62
Tangerines	1 large	40
Iron—Adult RDA = 10–18 mg		
Meats		
Calf liver, cooked	3-1/2 oz	12.4
Beef liver, cooked	3-1/2 oz	7.8
Chicken liver, cooked	2 livers	6.0
Beef, lean round, cooked	3-1/2 oz	3.5
Chicken, cooked, no bone	3-1/2 oz	2.1
Egg, boiled	1 medium	1.1
Fruits		
Watermelon	1/16 melon (10 × 16)	4.5
Prunes	8 large	4.4
Dates, dried	1/4 cup	1.4
Apricots, dried	4 halves	1.4
Raisins	1/4 cup	1.3
Blueberries, raw	1 cup	1.0
Strawberries, raw	10 large	1.0
Vegetables		
Spinach, raw	3-1/2 oz	3.1
Beans, cooked		

		mg/Portion
Kidney	1/2 cup	3.0
White	1/2 cup	2.7
Lima	1/2 cup	2.0
Asparagus, canned	5–6 medium	2.0
Lettuce, iceberg	1/4 head	2.0
Spinach, cooked	1/2 cup	2.0
Mustard Greens, cooked	1/2 cup	1.8
Green peas, cooked	1/2 cup	1.4
Cauliflower, raw	1 cup	1.1
Miscellaneous		
Molasses, medium	1 tbsp	1.2

Phosphorus—Adult RDA = 800 mg

		mg/Portion
Meats		
Calf liver, cooked	3-1/2 oz	537
Cod, broiled	3-1/2 oz	274
Beef, lean round, cooked	3-1/2 oz	250
Pork, lean, cooked	3-1/2 oz	249
Halibut, broiled	3-1/2 oz	248
Dairy Products		
Milk, whole	1 cup	227
Cheese		
Swiss	1 oz	158
Cottage, creamed	1/3 cup	152
Cheddar	1 oz	134

(Continued)

Appendix H—Continued

Food	Portion Size	Amount of Mineral
Brick	1 oz	127
Blue or Roquefort	1 oz	95
Nuts		
Peanuts, roasted	3 tbsp	180
Brazil	4 nuts	104
Peanut Butter	1 tbsp	59
Vegetables		
Beans, cooked		
Kidney	1/2 cup	175
White	1/2 cup	148
Lima	1/2 cup	97
Green peas, fresh, cooked	1/2 cup	75
Artichokes, cooked	1 bud	69
Potatoes, white, baked	1 small	65
Brussels sprouts, cooked	1/2 cup	55
Miscellaneous	10 oz	2–47
Zinc— Adult RDA = 15 mg		**mg/Portion**
Meats		
Oysters, Atlantic, raw	5–8 medium	160
Oysters, Pacific, raw	6–9 medium	31
Beef liver	3-1/2 oz	3.0–8.5

Eggs	1 egg	2.8
Beef	3-1/2 oz	2–5
Clams	4 large/9 small	2.0
Vegetables		
Corn	1/2 cup	3.1
Beets	2 beets	2.8
Peas	1/2 cup	2.3–3.8
Carrots	1/2 cup	0.4–2.7
Spinach	1/2 cup	0.3–0.8
Cabbage	1/2 cup	0.1–0.8
Lettuce	1/4 head	0.1–0.7
Cereal products		
Barley	1/2 cup	0.6
Bread, whole wheat	1 slice	0.7–1.0
Bread, rye	1 slice	0.5
Fruits		
Cherries, canned	1/2 cup	1.6–2.2
Pears, canned	2 small halves	1.5–1.8

SOURCE: Krause, Marie V. and Kathleen L. Mahan *Food, Nutrition and Diet Therapy: A Textbook of Nutritional Care,* 7th Edition. W.B. Saunders Co., 1984. Used with permission.

Foods with Special Implications for the Person with a Gastrointestinal Stoma

Bulk-Forming Foods

Celery
Chinese Food
Foods with seeds or kernels
Nuts
Coleslaw
Dried Fruits
Coconut
Wild Rice
Popcorn
Meats in casings
Whole Vegetables
Whole Grains

Odor-Causing Foods

Fish
Eggs
Asparagus
Onions
Garlic
Some Spices
Peas
Beans
Cabbage
Broccoli
Turnips

Diarrhea-Causing Foods

Green Beans
Broccoli
Spinach
Raw fruits
Highly seasoned foods

Gas-Forming Foods

String Beans
Dried Beans
Mushrooms
Carbonated Beverages, Beer
Dairy Products

(Continued)

Appendix I—Continued

Diarrhea-Causing Foods (*Cont.*)	Gas-Forming Foods (*Cont.*)
Beer (other alcoholic beverages are not common offenders	Cucumbers
	Onions
	Brussel Sprouts
	Peas
	Corn
	Broccoli
	Cauliflower
	Spinach
	Cabbage
	Radishes
	Yeast

Reproduced by permission from Hunker, Edith M.; *Nutrition Therapy for the Ostomy Patient.* In Broadwell, Debra C., and Jackson, Bettie S., editors: "Principles of Ostomy Care," St. Louis, 1982, The C. V. Mosby Co.

Nutritional Formulas and Preparations Commonly Available

Product Name/ Company	Sizes Available (oz, ctn)	Serving Size
Liquids		
Ensure/Ross	8-, 14-, 32-oz cans	8 oz
Ensure Plus/Ross	8-oz can or bottle	8 oz
Isocal/Mead Johnson	8-, 12- or 32-oz can	8 oz
Isocal HCN/Mead Johnson	8-oz can	8 oz
Isomil/Ross	13-oz can concentrated 8-, 32-oz can dilute	10 oz
Magnacal/Organon	250-cc bottle	8 oz
Meritene/Doyle	8-oz can	8 oz
Nutri-1000/Cutler	32-oz can	10 oz
Nutri-1000LF/Cutler	32-oz can	10 oz
Prosobee/[ab] Mead Johnson	13-oz can concentrate 8-, 32-oz read to use	10 oz
Sustacal/[a] Mead Johnson	8-, 12-oz can	8 oz
Sustacal HC/Mead Johnson	8-oz can	8 oz

Approximate Content per Serving		Special Considerations	Flavors Available
Calories	Protein (gm)		
250	8.8	Lactose and milk free, contains soy protein	Vanilla, strawberry egg nog, chocolate, black walnut, coffee
355	13.0	Lactose and milk free, contains soy protein	Vanilla, coffee, egg nog, strawberry, chocolate
250	8.1	Lactose and milk free, contains blend of soy and MCT oil	Mild taste, unflavored
473	17.7	Lactose and milk free, contains blend of soy and MCT oil	Mild taste, unflavored
200	6.0	Lactose and milk free, contains soy protein	
480	17.0	Lactose and milk free	Vanilla
300	18.0	Contains milk	Vanilla, chocolate, egg nog
313	11.3	Contains milk	Vanilla, chocolate
313	11.3	Lactose free, contains soy protein	
200	5.9	Contains soy protein isolate, Lactose free, sucrose-free	
240	14.5	Contains soy protein isolate and caseinates, lactose-free	Vanilla, Chocolate, egg nog
360	14.4	Lactose free	Vanilla, egg nog

(Continued)

Appendix J—Continued

Product Name/ Company	Sizes Available (oz, ctn)	Serving Size
Powders [c]		
Citrotein/Doyle	12-oz can	6 oz
	1.18-oz packets	
Instant Breakfast, Carnation	Ctn of 6, 1.26-oz packets	1 packet
Meritene/Doyle	1-lb can	1.14 oz measure
Sustacal/[ab] Mead Johnson	Ctn of 4, 1.9-oz packets 3.8-lb. can	1 packet
Sustagen/Mead Johnson		2/3 cup packed
Pudding		
Forta/Ross	5-oz can	5 oz
Sustacal/[a] Mead Johnson	5-oz can	5 oz

[a] Recipes available from the manufacturer
[b] Available where infant formulas are sold
[c] Calorie and protein content when prepared as directed on the package
Source: U.S. Department of Health and Human Services, Public Health Service, NIH, *Eating Hints—Recipes and Tips for Better Nutrition During Cancer Treatment.*

Note: All Supplements should be checked with the physician before using to be sure they are compatible with other medications.

Approximate Content per Serving		Special Considerations	Flavors Available
127	7.7	Lactose free, contains egg whites	Orange, grape, fruit punch
290	16.0	Contains milk and soy protein, high lactose	6 flavors
277	18.0	Contains milk, high lactose	Vanilla, chocolate, egg nog
360	20.5	Contains milk, high lactose	Vanilla, chocolate, egg nog
390	23.5	Low fat, contains lactose	Vanilla, chocolate
250	6.8	Low lactose	Vanilla, chocolate, tapioca and butterscotch
240	6.8	Low lactose contains milk	vanilla, chocolate, butterscotch

K

Drug/Nutrient Interactions

Therapeutic Class	Drug Name		Recommended Daily Vitamin/Mineral Supplement or Restriction During Drug Therapy[a]
	Proprietary Examples	Generic/Active Compound	
Dermatological preparation	Accutane	isotretinoin	Avoid Vitamin A Supplement
Antibiotics	Panmycin Achromycin Other Aureomycin	tetracycline chlortetracycline	Riboflavin (B2), 5 mg Ascorbic Acid, 100–200 mg; Calcium, 0.8–1.5 gm[b]
Anticonvulsants	Dilantin	phenytoin	Vitamin D, 400–800 IU[c] Vitamin K, 1–5 mg Folic Acid, 0.4–1.0 mg (not >2.0 mg/day)
	Mysoline	primidone	Vitamin K, 1–5 mg[c]
Anti-inflammatory	Azulfidine Bayer Aspirin Bufferin Other Aspirin Indocin	sulfasalazine aspirin indomethacin	Folic acid, 0.4–1.0 mg Ascorbic acid, 50–100 mg, Folic Acid, 0.4–1.0 mg Iron, 20–50 mg Iron, 20–50 mg
Antilipemic	Questran	cholestyramine	Vitamin A, 2000–5000 IU

(Continued)

Appendix K—Continued

Therapeutic Class	Drug Name		Recommended Daily Vitamin/Mineral Supplement or Restriction During Drug Therapy[a]
	Proprietary Examples	Generic/Active Compound	
	Colestid	colestipol	Vitamin D, 200–800 IU Vitamin K, 2–25 mg[d] Folic Acid, 0.4–1.0 mg
Antituberculous	INH Rifamate	isoniazid rifampin-isoniazid	Vitamin B$_6$, 25–50 mg Niacin, 15–25 mg Vitamin D, 400–800 IU
Anticoagulant	Coumadin	coumarin anticoagulants	Avoid Vitamin K
Diuretic	Dyrenium Dyazide	triamterene	Folic Acid, 0.4–1.0 mg
Gastrointestinal	Agoral	mineral oil	Vitamin A, 5000–10,000 IU[e] Vitamin D, 400–800 IU Folic Acid, 0.4–1 mg
	Soda Mint	antacids	
Hypotensive	Apresoline	hydralazine	Vitamin B$_6$, 25–100 mg
Oral contraceptives	Norinyl	estrogen/progestin	Vitamin B$_6$, 1.5–5 mg

		Demulen Ovral Ortho-Novum Modicon and others	Folic Acid, 0.4–1 mg Avoid high doses of Vitamin C (anything >1000 mg)
Tranquilizer	chloropromazine thioridazine other phenothiazines	Thorazine Mellaril	Riboflavin, 2–5 mg
Other	levodopa penicillamine	Larodopa Depen	Vitamin B₆, restrict supplement <5 mg Vitamin B6, 25–100 mg

a Short-term drug therapy may or may not necessitate specific vitamin/mineral supplementation.

b Calcium-containing foods and supplements should be given > 2 hours away from drug dose.

c If Dilantin (phenytoin)-induced demineralization is identified, give Vitamin D 2000 IU/day. Pregnant women on Dilantin or Mysoline should receive Vitamin K, 5 mg/day for 3 days prior to delivery and neonate should receive 1 mg.

d Routine use of Vitamin K, not required with Questran (cholestyramine) or Colestid (colestipol). Give Vitamin K1 I.M. in stated dosage range if hypoprothrombinemia exists

e When daily dose of mineral oil preparation equals or exceeds 30 mL/day, a vitamin supplement is required. Mineral oil should be taken at bedtime and never within 2 hours of a meal.

NOTE: Pregnant or lactating women should consult their physicians for specific micronutrient recommendations.

Prepared by Daphne Roe, M.D., Professor of Nutrition, Cornell University, Ithaca, New York, as a service to the health profession by Hoffmann-LaRoche, Inc. Used With Permission.

L

Drug-Induced Coloration of the Urine

Many drugs have been reported to cause discoloration of body excreta. Discolored urine may cause undue anxiety in patients and failure to take prescribed drugs.

Discoloration is usually dependent on the concentration of the drug in the urine and on the concentration of the urine itself. It can be helpful to caution patients about this potential drug-induced urine discoloration.

Type	Drug	Color of Urine
Analgesics	Phenacetin	Dark brown
	Salicylates	Pink to brown (due to bleeding)
	Indocin (Indomethacin)	Green (due to biliverdinemia)
Analgesics, Urinary	Pyridium (Phenazophridine)	Red-orange
		Often stains permanently
Anticoagulants		Dark red (due to bleeding)
Anticonvulsants	Dilantin (diphenylhydantoin)	Pink to red-brown
	Milontin (phensuximide)	Pink to red-brown
Antidepressants	Elavil, Endep (amitriptyline)	Blue-green
Anti-infectives	Quinine and derivatives	Brown to black
	Atabrine (quinacrine)	Yellow
	Flagyl (metronidazole)	Dark
	Nitrofurans	Yellow to brown
	Rifadin, Rimactane, (rifampin)	Red-orange
	Sulfonamides	Yellow to brown

(Continued)

Appendix L—Continued

Type	Drug	Color of Urine
Antiparkinsonian	Dopar, Laradopa (levodopa)	Darkens on standing
	Sinemet (metoclopramide)	Darkens on standing
Diuretics	Dyrenium (triamterene)	Pale blue
Hematinics	Iron-Salts	Dark
Laxatives	Cascara	Red
	Phenolphthalein	Red
	Antihraquinones	Pink to brown
	Senna	Red in alkaline urine, Yellow-brown in acid urine
Muscle Relaxants	Paraflex (chlorzoxazone)	Purple to orange
	Robaxin (methocarbamol)	Brown to black, green on standing
Tranquilizers	Phenothiazines	Pink to brown
Vitamins	Riboflavin	Yellow
Miscellaneous	Desferal (deferoxamine)	Reddish
	Methylene blue	Green to blue

M

Selected Ostomy Skin Sealants and Barriers

Appendix M—Continued

	Preparations	Characteristics
Orabase	**Paste** made of gelatin, pectin, and sodium carboxymethylcellulose in a polyethylene and mineral oil gel base; sensitivities rare.	Adheres tenaciously to moist surfaces, either normal or eroded skin; does not cause pain when applied; melts or washes away more rapidly than Stomahesive.
Stomahesive	**Solid Wafers** 4 × 4 or 8 × 8 in. made of gelatin, pectin, sodium carboxymethylcellulose, and polyisobutylene laminated between polyethylene film and an opaque backing of paper; sensitivities rare.	Adheres to normal, erythematous, moist, or eroded skin; does not cause pain when applied; an effective skin barrier available in solid form; does not melt readily with heat; paste contains alcohol.
	Powder or Paste made of gelatin, pectin, and sodium carboxymethylcellulose; sensitivities rare.	Adheres to normal, erythematous, moist, or eroded skin; powder does not cause pain when applied.
Karaya Powder	**Powder** a naturally occuring gum and a partially acetylated polysaccharide; comes in plastic bottles or shaker-top cans or jars; sensitivities common.	Adheres to moist skin; will not adhere to dry skin; does not cause pain when applied to normal skin; causes burning, stinging pain when applied to irritated or eroded skin so should only be used on normal or slightly reddened skin.
Karaya washers or rings	**Solid Washers or Rings** light to dark brown in or rings color; comes in various diameters and thicknesses; can be obtained separately or attached to appliances; is a partially acetylated polysaccharide mixed with glycerine; sensitivities common.	Adheres to dry or moist skin; causes burning, stinging pain when applied to irritated or eroded skin so should be used only on normal or slightly reddened skin.

HolliHesive	**Solid Wafers** 4 × 4 or 8 × 8 in.; composition unknown; sensitivities rare.	Adheres to normal, erythematous, moist, or eroded skin; does not cause pain when applied; an effective skin barrier available in solid form; does not melt readily with heat.
Surgical Cement	**Liquid** made of latex and latex solvents; may contain zinc oxide; sensitivities common.	Used on normal, intact, dry skin; will not adhere to moist, irritated skin; must be left to dry (2–4 min) so solvents can evaporate.
Tincture of Benzoin	**Liquid** made of 10% benzoin and 90% alcohol; benzoin is balsamic resin from stem of a tree; (styrax); is ground and combined with alcohol; sensitivities common, particularly to compound tincture of benzoin, which contains storax, tolubalms, and aloes.	May be used only on intact normal skin; if applied to reddened or weeping skin, causes pain and more irritation and weeping of skin. On normal skin, increases adhesiveness of appliance and protects skin from irritation from adhesives.
Skin Gel	**Liquid or Spray** containing N-butyl/isobutyl methacrylate 50/50 copolymer, dimethylphthalate, glycerine, methylparaben, allantoin, and isopropyl alcohol; sensitivities rare.	May only be used on intact skin; if applied to reddened, eroded skin, exacerbates the condition. On normal skin provides a protective covering so that adhesives on appliances cause less irritation.
Skin Prep	**Liquid or Spray** containing vinyl resin, isopropyl alcohol, and dimethylphthalate; sensitivities rare.	May only be used on normal intact skin; if applied to reddened or eroded skin, causes pain and exacerbates the condition; on normal skin, provides a protective barrier that decreases incidence of irritation from appliance adhesives.
Soap and Water	**Solid Bar or Liquid** a mixture of fats and alkalis; many have scents and other additives; sensitivities infrequent.	Should be used only on normal skin; a noncreamy-based soap does not leave an oily residue on skin, which prevents adherence of adhesives; avoid Phisohex or Phisoderm.

(Continued)

Appendix M—Continued

	Preparations	Characteristics
Karaya Paste	**Paste** in 2-oz and 4-oz tubes; made of karaya, bantrez resin, isopropyl alcohol, and parasepts; occasional sensitivities.	Will adhere to dry skin only will not adhere to moist surfaces; if applied in layers thicker than 0.5 cm, will "drag;" with gravity; very painful when applied to irritated or eroded skin; very useful to fill in uneven contours on abdomen.
Crixiline	8×8 or 4×4 in. squares; rings are of various diameters; a blend of polyacrylamides with binding agents; sensitivities rare.	Seals well and forms a soft, cushiony pad; melts as rapidly as karaya; mineral oil will remove it from faceplates.
ReliaSeal	**Solid Rings or Washers** with various inside diameter openings; a pectin-based substance; sensitivities rare.	Works exceptionally well with urinary diversion; material swells with urine but skin remains normal; adheres best to dry skin but will adhere to moist, irritated skin; does not mold to body contours as well as Stomahesive or karaya.
Aluminum Paste	**Metallic Aluminum Powder** blended with zinc oxide ointment; sensitivities rare.	Messy paste that only adheres to dry skin; difficult to remove and clings to bed linens and other inappropriate areas; can be removed with mineral oil.

Reproduced by permission from Watt, Rosemary C. In Broadwell, Debra C. and Jackson, Bettie S., editors: "Principles of Ostomy Care," St. Louis, 1982, The C.V. Mosby Company.

N

Nursing Assessment Guide for Fluid and Electrolyte Status

Appendix N—Continued

Body area/system	Assessment	Reason
Weight		
Variations	% Loss (in lb):	
	< 5	Mild dehydration
	5–10	Moderate dehydration
	> 15	Severe dehydration
(In average size adult)	% Gain (in lbs):	
	< 5	Mild overhydration
	5–10	Moderate overhydration
	> 15	Severe overhydration
HEENT		
Eyes	Dry conjunctiva	Fluid volume deficit
	Decreased tearing	Fluid volume deficit
	Periorbital edema	Fluid volume excess
	Sunken	Fluid volume deficit
Mouth	Sticky, dry mucous membranes	Fluid volume deficit
	Increased viscosity saliva	Sodium excess
Lips	Dry, cracked	Sodium deficit
Tongue	Longitudinal furrows	Fluid volume deficit
		Sodium deficit
Cardiopulmonary		
Cardiovascular	Increased pulse rate	Fluid volume deficit
	Decreased pulse rate	Fluid volume deficit
	Bounding pulse	Fluid volume excess

System	Signs/Symptoms	Associated Imbalance
Respiratory	Decreased blood pressure	Fluid volume deficit
	Narrow pulse pressure	Fluid volume deficit
	Cardiac arrhythmias	Potassium deficit
	Jugular vein distension	Fluid volume excess
	Moist rales, rhonchi	Fluid volume excess
	Increased respiratory rate	Fluid volume excess
	Dyspnea	Fluid volume excess
	Pulmonary edema	Fluid volume excess
	Shallow, slow breathing	Metabolic alkalosis
	Respiratory acidosis	Metabolic acidosis
	Deep, rapid breathing	Respiratory alkalosis
Gastrointestinal	Abdominal cramps	Potassium excess
	Nausea, vomiting, diarrhea	Magnesium excess
Renal	Oliguria	Sodium deficit or excess
Extremities	Edema of dependent body parts such as sacrum, lower extremities	Fluid volume excess
Integumentary		
Temperature	Increased	Sodium excess
	Decreased	Fluid volume deficit
Skin Surfaces	Decreased turgor	Fluid volume deficit
	Warm, moist	Fluid volume excess
	Flushing	Magnesium deficit
Neurologic	Depressed CNS activity	Fluid volume deficit
	Increased Intracranial Pressure	Sodium deficit

(Continued)

Appendix N—Continued

Body area/system	Assessment	Reason
Musculoskeletal	Positive Babinski's sign	Magnesium deficit
	Disorientation or confusion	Acidosis or alkalosis
	Muscle weakness	Potassium deficit
		Calcium excess
	Hypertonus:	Calcium deficit
	Positive Chvostek's Sign	Metabolic alkalosis
	Carpopedal spasm	Calcium deficit
		Metabolic alkalosis
	Muscle rigidity	Muscle alkalosis

Reprinted with permission from the March issue of Nursing 82, Copyright Springhouse Corporation, all rights reserved.

Equivalent Measures

Weights

Apothecary	Metric	Apothecary	Metric
1 ounce	= 31.1 gm	1/150 grain =	0.4 mg
15.43 grains	= 1 gm	1/200 grain =	0.3 mg
1 grain	= 60 mg	1/250 grain =	0.25 mg
1/60 grain	= 1.0 mg	1/300 grain =	0.2 mg
1/80 grain	= 0.8 mg	1/400 grain =	0.15 mg
1/100 grain	= 0.6 mg	1/500 grain =	0.12 mg
1/120 grain	= 0.5 mg	1/600 grain =	0.1 mg

Liquid Measure

Household	Apothecary	Approximate Metric
1 teaspoonful	1 fluid dram	5 mL
1 dessertspoonful	2 fluid drams	8 mL
1 tablespoonful	4 fluid drams	15 mL
2 tablespoonfuls	1 fluid oz	30 mL
1 measuring cupful	8 fluid oz	240 mL
1 jigger	1½ fluid oz	45 mL
1 wineglassful	2 fluid oz	60 mL
1 teacupful	4 fluid oz	120 mL
1 glassful	8 fluid oz	240 mL
1 pint	16 fluid oz	500 mL
1 quart	32 fluid oz	1000 mL

Temperature

$$9 \ (°C) \ - \ = 5 \ (°F) \ - \ 160$$
$$(°C \times 9/5) + 32 = °F$$
$$(°F - 32) \times 5/9 = °C$$

(Continued)

Appendix O—Continued

Metric Weight Equivalents

1 kg = 1,000 gm
1 gm = 1,000 mg
1 mg = 0.001 gm
1 mcg or μg = 0.001 mg

Conversions

1 oz = 30 gm
1 lb = 453.6 gm
2.2 lb = 1 kg

Metric Volume Equivalents

1 liter = 1,000 mL
1 deciliter = 100 mL

Bibliography

General

Beare, Patricia Gauntlett, et. al. *Quick Reference To Nursing Implications of Diagnostic Tests.* Philadelphia: J.B. Lippincott Company, 1983.

Govoni, Laura E. and Janice E. Hayes *Drugs and Nursing Implications, Fourth Edition.* Norwalk, Conn.: Appleton-Century-Crofts, 1982.

Holloway, Vonicha McClenny *Home Healthcare Nurse,* January/February, 1984, 19–20.

Hoole, Axalla, et. al. *Patient Care Guidelines for Nurse Practitioners, Second Edition.* Boston: Little, Brown and Company, 1982.

Jaffe, Marie S. and Linda C. Skidmore *Diagnostic and Laboratory Cards for Clinical Use.* Bowie, Md.: Robert J. Brady Company, 1984.

Keithley, Joyce and Kay Fraulini *Nursing 82,* 12, No. 3 (March 1982), 33–42.

Kilo, Carles *Educating the Diabetic Patient.* New York: Pfizer Laboratories, 1982.

Metheny, Norma Mulligan and W.D. Snively *Nurses' Handbook of Fluid Balance, Fourth Edition.* Philadelphia: J.B. Lippincott Company, 1983.

Nursing 83 Books Staff *Procedures, Nurses Reference Library Series.* Springhouse, Penn.: Nursing '83 Books, 1983.

Shamansky, Sherry, M. Carolyn Cecere, Evelyn Shellenberger *Primary Health Care Handbook.* Boston: Little, Brown and Company, 1984.

Steiger, Nancy J. and Juliene G. Lipson *Self-Care Nursing: Theory and Practice.* Bowie, Md.: Brady Communications Company, Inc., 1985.

Assessment

Bates, Barbara *A Guide to Physical Examination, Third Edition.* Philadelphia: J.B. Lippincott Co., 1983.

DeGowin, Elmer L. and Richard L. DeGowin *Bedside Diagnositc Examination, Fourth Edition.* New York: Macmillan Publishing Company, Inc., 1981.

Kastrup, Erwin K. and James R. Boyd *Facts and Comparisons*. Philadelphia: J.B. Lippincott Company, 1985.

Lynch, Peter J. *Dermatology for the House Officer*. Baltimore: Williams and Wilkins, 1982.

Malasanos, Lois, et. al. *Health Assessment, Second Edition*. St. Louis: The C.V. Mosby, Company, 1981.

Nursing 83 Books Staff *Assessment, Nurses Reference Library Series*. Springhouse, Penn.: Nursing '83 Books, 1983.

Rudy, Ellen and V. Ruth Gray *Handbook of Health Assessment*. Bowie, Md.: Robert J. Brady Company, 1981.

Interventions

Brunner, Lillian and Doris Suddarth *The Lippincott Manual of Nursing Practice, Third Edition*. Philadelphia: J.B. Lippincott Company, 1982.

Covell, Mara *The Home Alternative to Hospitals & Nursing Homes*. New York: Rawson Associates, 1983.

Cancer

DeVita, V.T., H. Hillman, and S.A. Rosenberg, *Cancer: Principles and Practices of Oncology, 2nd Edition*. Philadelphia: J.B. Lippincott Company, 1985.

Dilworth, John A. and Gerald L. Mandell *Seminars in Oncology*, Vol. 2, No. 4 (December), 1975, 349–356.

Donovan, Constance T. *Infection Control and Urological Care*, Vol.7, No. 2, 1982, 27–30.

Johnson, Bonny L. and Jody Gross *Handbook of Oncology Nursing*. New York: John Wiley & Sons, 1985.

Morra, Marion and Eve Potts *Choices: Realistic Alternatives In Cancer Treatment*. New York: Avon Books, 1980.

Sickles, Edward, et. al. *Archives of Internal Medicine*, Vol. 135, (May) 1975, 715–719.

Yasko, Joyce M. *Guidelines for Cancer Care Symptom Management*. Reston, Va.: Reston Publishing Company, 1983.

Wound Care

Broadwell, Debra and Bettie Jackson *Principles of Ostomy Care*. St. Louis: The C.V. Mosby Company, 1982.

Cooper, Diane M., et. al. *Guide to Wound Care*. Liberty-ville, Ill.: Hollister Incorporated, 1983.

Hunt, et al. *Wound Healing & Wound Infection: Theory and Surgical Practice*. Norwalk, Conn.: Appleton-Century-Crofts, 1980.

Peacock, E.E. and W. VanWinkle, *Wound Repair, Second Edition*. Philadelphia: W.B. Saunders Company, 1976.

Mental Status—Cognitive Functioning

Hall, Richard *Manifestations of Medical Illness: Somatopsychic Disorders*. New York: S.P. Medical and Scientific Books, 1980.

American Psychiatric Association, *Quick Reference to the Diagnositc Criteria from DSM-III*. Washington, D.C., 1980.

Levy, Ronald, M.D. *The New Language of Psychiatry: Learning and Using DSM III*. Boston: Little, Brown and Company, 1982.

Nutrition—Diet

American Dietetic Association *Handbook of Clinical Dietetics*. New Haven, Conn.: Yale University Press, 1981.

Applied Nutrition in Clinical Medicine *The Medical Clinics of North America*, Vol. 63, No. 5. Philadelphia: W.B. Saunders, Company, 1979.

Berland, T. *Rating the Diets, Consumer Guide*. New York: Signet Books, 1979.

Krause, Marie V. and L. Kathleen Mahan *Food, Nutrition, and Diet Therapy: A Textbook of Nutritional Care, Seventh Edition*. Philadelphia: W.B. Saunders Company, 1984.

Morra, M., N. Suski, B. Johnson *Eating Hints: Recipes and Tips For Better Nutrition During Cancer Therapy*. Bethesda, Md.: National Cancer Institute, (NIH Pub. No. 82-2079), 1982.

U.S. Government Printing Office *Nutritive Value of American Foods*, Agriculture Handbook 456. Washington, D.C., 1975.

Wilford, L. *Nutritive Value of Convenience Foods, Third Edition* Hines, Ill.: West Surburban Dietetic Association, 1982.

Nutrition—Cookbooks

American Heart Association *Cooking Without Your Salt Shaker*. Dallas, Tex.: AHA, 1978. (Copies may be purchased at local affiliates.)

Middleton, K. and M. Hess *The Art of Cooking for the Diabetic*. Boston: CBI Publishing Company, Inc., 1974.

Nonken, P. and R. Hirsch *The Allergy Cookbook and Food-Buying Guide*. New York: Warner Books, Inc., 1982.

Robertson, L., C. Flinders, B. Godfrey *Laurel's Kitchen*. New New York: Bantam Books, 1978.

Community Health Nursing Textbooks

Leahy, Kathleen, M. Marguerite Cobb, Mary Jones *Community Health Nursing, Second Edition*. New York: McGraw-Hill Book Company, 1972.

Burgess, Wendy and Ethel Chatterton Ragland *Community Health Nursing—Philosophy, Process, Practice*. Norwalk, Conn.: Appleton-Century-Crofts, 1983.

Spradley, Barbara Walton *Community Health Nursing—Concepts and Practice*. Boston: Little, Brown and Company, 1981.

Stanhope, Marcia and Jeanette Lancaster *Community Health Nursing Process and Practice for Promoting Health*. St. Louis: The C.V. Mosby Company, 1984.

Elkins, Carolyn Pinion *Community Health Nursing—Skills and Strategies*. Bowie, Md.: Robert J. Brady Company, 1984.

Index

Your Own Pages

Your Own Pages

Your Own Pages

Your Own Pages

Your Own Pages

Your Own Pages

Your Own Pages